The
PHYSICIAN'S
OFFICE
LABORATORY

The
PHYSICIAN'S OFFICE LABORATORY

Richard E. Belsey, MD

Head of Chemical Pathology Division,
Professor of Clinical Pathology, Asssociate
Professor of Medicine, Oregon Health
Sciences University, Portland

Daniel M. Baer, MD

Chief of Laboratory Service, VA Medical
Center, Professor of Clinical Pathology,
Oregon Health Sciences University, Portland

Bernard E. Statland, MD, PhD

Director of Laboratory Medicine, University
Hospital, Boston; Professor of Pathology,
Medicine, and Biochemistry, Boston
University Medical School

David L. Sewell, PhD

Section Director of Microbiology, VA
Medical Center, Portland; Associate Professor
of Clinical Pathology, Oregon Health
Sciences University, Portland

Medical Economics Books
Oradell, N.J. 07649

Library of Congress Cataloging in Publication Data

Belsey, Richard E.
   The physician's office laboratory.

   Includes index.
   1. Diagnosis, Laboratory.   2. Medical laboratories—
Management.   3. Diagnosis, Laboratory—Economic
aspects.   I. Baer, Daniel M., 1931-   .   II. Statland,
Bernard E.   III. Title.   [DNLM: 1. Diagnosis, Laboratory
—methods.   2. Diagnostic Tests, Routine.   3. Health
Facilities—organization & administration.   4. Labora-
tories—organization & administration.   QY   23   B452p]
RB37.B444   1986   616.07'5   86-5196
ISBN 0-87489-408-5 (soft)

Art Director Penina M. Wissner
Interior design by Penny Seldin
Cover design by Sharyn Banks

ISBN 0-87489-408-5

Medical Economics Company Inc.
Oradell, New Jersey 07649

Printed in the United States of America

To Monroe Mendelsohn, a colleague and friend, who was, in the last year of his life, a catalyst bringing a new perspective that stimulated us to look at the world in fresh and innovative ways.

Table of contents

PART II   ECONOMICS AND REGULATORY FOUNDATIONS

PART III   THE ANALYTICAL PRACTICE OF OFFICE TESTING

Preface

In a sense, laboratory testing has come full circle. Years ago, most physicians did a substantial amount of testing in their offices. Then came the development of big, fast instruments that provided many results from a small specimen at a low unit cost. The machines themselves were expensive, however, and required highly skilled technologists to operate them, so centralized testing became the mode. It was accurate, carefully controlled, and cost-effective; and testing in other sites such as the physician's office diminished markedly.

Now, technology has once again made it possible for the physician to perform a variety of clinically useful test analyses in the office laboratory. Today's new test systems are inexpensive and relatively simple to operate. Employees without formal laboratory training can quickly produce accurate results for immediate use in patient care.

Although many laboratorians are concerned about testing leaving the laboratory, they must admit that the new technology has made test results available when and where it counts—in the physician's office or at the bedside in hospitals' critical care areas. Removing analysis from these settings was important at first, as it provided an expanded menu of accurate tests for diagnosing and managing patient problems. But it quickly became apparent that the initial methods used on the large analyzers (adapted from old manual methods) were imprecise and often inaccurate. Over the past three decades, the advances in laboratory quality assurance have provided a foundation for the current high quality of laboratory practice.

We are particularly concerned over this issue of quality assurance. We believe that while the new technology will facilitate and improve patient care in the office practice, it carries potential hazards. The practitioner must be aware of underlying complexities. Although superficially simple to use (almost as easy as a television set), the test procedures involve complex analytic systems. Whoever is professionally responsible for the office laboratory—usually the physician—should have some understanding of these complexities. Each office laboratory should be able to document the validity and reliability of the test results on a day-to-day basis. The physician and the laboratory staff should also consult professional laboratorians in the community for help with problems that are beyond their competence.

This book is designed to assist practitioners who already have office laboratories and to serve as an introduction to those who are thinking about starting one. It will also be useful for medical students and house staff in understanding the issues involved in analysis and applying test results to patient care. Part I addresses the clinical aspects of office laboratory medicine, including the selection of appropriate testing and the interpretation of lab results. The office context differs from that of the hospital. In the former, most patients walk in with common, nonspecific symptoms. An immediate understanding of the patient's problem is often elusive, and the practitioner considers the use of diagnostic tests, special studies, consultation, or simply waiting. The hospitalized patient is already defined as being sick; the need is to differentiate various diagnoses in order to embark on the appropriate treatment course.

The selection, use, and interpretation of office laboratory testing can be important in the physician-patient relationship as well as in the diagnostic process. We look at these issues, too, including some selected clinical problems. Economic and regulatory considerations also figure in the decision to bring test analysis into the office laboratory. Part II contains a discussion of cost accounting for the laboratory and an introduction to reimbursement issues. Regulation of physicians' office laboratories is primarily a responsibility of the states, and, as we point out, the rules vary widely. In addition, office testing increases physicians' tort liability exposure; in this section of the book, we show how to minimize the risk of such liability.

Once the decision has been made to perform office testing, the physician needs guidance in setting up the laboratory, selecting personnel, and developing safety protocols in what will probably be the most hazardous area in the office. Part III deals with these issues and describes the various methods and systems available, providing guidelines for selecting systems and supervising patients' self-testing. In the discussion of quality assurance, we stress the importance of documenting the validity and reliability of laboratory test results and provide tips on how to select reference laboratories and best use these consultants.

Publisher's notes

If you are now doing office testing, or are measuring the feasibility and means of starting a laboratory, four leaders in clinical medicine and lab management here team up to help you take all the right steps to plan, finance, set up, operate, and monitor an effective and efficient lab in your office.

Richard E. Belsey, MD, is head of chemical pathology and professor of clinical pathology and medicine at Oregon Health Sciences University in Portland, and editor of *Office Lab Letter,* published by American Health Consultants in Atlanta.

Daniel M. Baer, MD, is chief of laboratory service at the VA Medical Center in Portland, professor of clinical pathology at Oregon Health Sciences University, and editor of *Interpretations in Therapeutic Drug Monitoring* (1981), published by the American Society of Clinical Pathologists.

Bernard E. Statland, MD, PhD, is director of laboratory medicine at University Hospital in Boston, professor of pathology, medicine, and biochemistry at Boston University Medical School, author of *Clinical Decision Levels for Lab Tests* (1983), and editor of *DRG Survival Manual for the Clinical Lab* (1985), both published by Medical Economics Books.

David L. Sewell, PhD, is section director of microbiology at the VA Medical Center in Portland, and associate professor of clinical pathology at Oregon Health Sciences University.

ACKNOWLEDGMENTS

The authors gratefully acknowledge key contributions made by:

Shirley Bott, MT (ASCP), *on troubleshooting in Chapter 17*

Catherine Cohen, MA, *on regulation and reimbursement in Chapter 6*

Michael A. Greene, JD, *on liability in Chapter 7*

Terry Kenny, MT (ASCP), *on pregnancy testing in Chapter 15*

The clinical practice of office testing

1

The laboratory testing loop

Office laboratory testing must be considered in the context of the clinical problems the practitioner encounters. They are radically different from those in the hospital setting, where the concern is making the differential diagnosis and starting appropriate treatment in the acutely ill patient. In the office, most patients walk in with common, nonspecific complaints and symptoms that are often difficult to characterize. Consequently, a major question for the office practitioner is whether the presenting signs and symptoms are significant enough to justify classifying the patient as being sick.

The diagnostic process in the office is also quite different from that in the hospital or acute-care setting. With nonemergency office patients, diagnosis and management seek to reduce uncertainty and find a plausible explanation of the symptoms. The practitioner must also decide whether it's appropriate or necessary to control symptoms before making a definitive diagnosis.

The history and physical are of, course, the key elements of the office workup. A well-established doctor-patient relationship makes it easier to evaluate the information, which may well be modulated by the patient's personal style and health concerns. When the history and physical provide no clear indication of the underlying problem, additional options include laboratory tests, other diagnostic studies, and clinical consultation, each of which may be sought for a variety of reasons. Some are related to evalu-

3

ating the problem itself, others to the care of and relationship with the patient. The physician may use tests to document or define the nature of a problem or simply to temporize—to reassure the patient or enhance the patient-physician relationship. ("My doctor always does a laboratory test; that's good!"). When uncertain about the cause of a problem, the practitioner may find that ordering a test or procedure is often easier and less time-consuming than facing the uncertainty and sharing it with the patient.

It should be noted, incidentally, that laboratory testing or clinical consultation is not intrinsically positive or even neutral in the health-care process; it may actually have an adverse impact. Merely ordering a laboratory procedure, for example, can confirm the sick role in a patient's mind—regardless of its result. In addition, if tests are ordered to temporize, the patient and the practitioner may both stop thinking about the problem until the results are available; when they both might be better served by continuing the diagnostic process and further defining the medical history. Information on progressing or changing signs and symptoms can be quite relevant to understanding the problem. In the office setting even more than in the hospital, continued patient involvement in the information-gathering process can speed the diagnosis.

Uncertainty is a fact of life in the office practice, however. Managing a patient's problem almost always requires judgments based on inadequate information. In contrast to the hospital setting, where emergent problems often dictate immediate decisions, the office patient is usually physiologically (but not necessarily psychologically) well compensated. Consequently, management decisions can generally be deferred, while continuing to seek clues to the underlying cause of the problem.

It should be emphasized that the best way to define a patient's problem is with a thorough, ongoing process of gathering information. This embraces taking the medical history, assessing life-style (alcoholism is best diagnosed this way—see Chapter 5), recording symptoms of affective disorders, inquiring about such support networks as family and friends, and learning the patient's own concerns and beliefs about health. This is best done in the office, where developing trust can provide the basis for superior patient care.

The laboratory testing loop

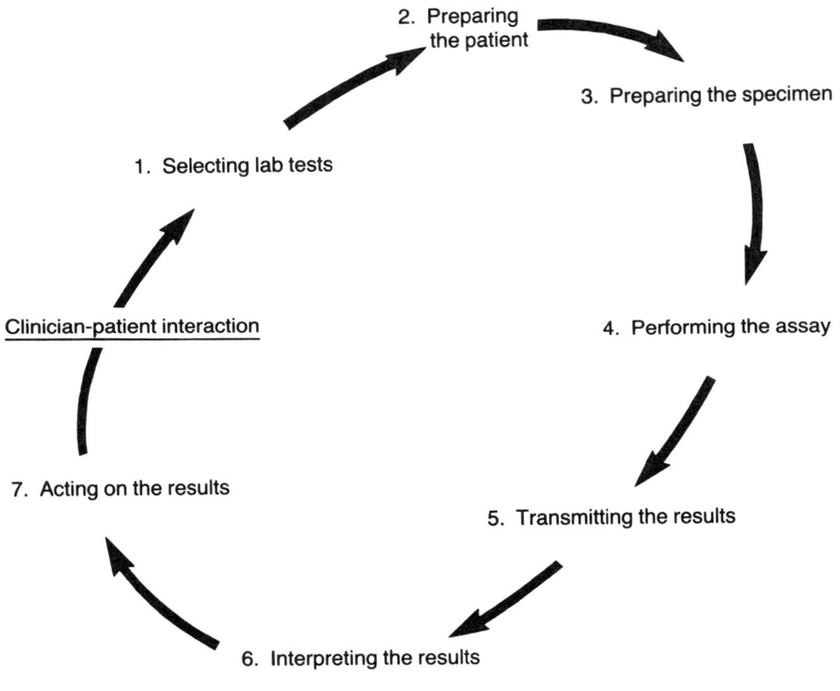

The preceding comments notwithstanding, laboratory tests can often be extremely useful in caring for the office patient. Using laboratory test results in diagnosis and management is a complex process that starts with the clinician-patient interaction but also involves a number of other obligatory steps in the laboratory testing loop (Figure 1-1).

This loop begins with the clinician-patient interaction, which can be initiated by the patient, the clinician, or a third party. The patient may seek care because of general health concerns or specific mental or physical symptoms. Alternatively, the clinician may ask the patient to return for further exploration of a problem. This might follow an unusual physical finding or laboratory result or something uncovered during screening. Finally, an employer, a government agency, an insurance company, or other third party may call for a medical examination as a prerequisite to employment, to issuing an insurance policy, or to documenting ongoing disability. Whatever the nature of the doctor-patient interaction, both parties need a satisfactory conclusion. When a third party is involved, it too must find the interaction acceptable.

In the past, most of a clinician's investigative and therapeutic decisions were made without laboratory testing. Today, however, physicians rely heavily on laboratory test information for diagnosing and managing patient problems. The sequence of events is shown in seven distinct steps of the testing loop, starting with test selection and ending with a decision based on its results.

The basic purpose of diagnostic testing is to put patients in appropriate clinical categories, while that of patient-management tests is to determine prognosis, response to therapy, or disease activity. We discuss the rationale and theoretical basis for requesting laboratory tests in terms of diagnostic sensitivity, specificity, and predictive value of positive or negative test results in Chapter 2.

Selecting the tests, insuring that the patient is properly prepared, interpreting the test result, and applying the information to patient management (steps 1, 2, 6, and 7 in the testing loop) have traditionally been the clinician's responsibilities. Chapter 3 discusses patient preparation before the specimen is collected, including dietary restrictions, drug ingestion, exercise, smoking, and posture.

Chapter 4, in which we discuss interpreting laboratory information, requires an understanding of the concept of normal, or reference, values. Laboratory values are usually interpreted in relationship to a group of peers (group-specific reference values) or in relationship to the patient's own previous values (patient-specific reference values). With some laboratory tests, demographic considerations such as age, pregnancy, sex, and race are significant variables and, therefore, must be considered when defining group-specific values. For patient-specific values, the importance of expected biologic variation of certain analytes within a single subject must be considered before applying test results to patient management decisions.

The final step in the testing loop is applying the information to patient-care problems. The physician might then make a prognostic decision, such as whether to share the prognosis with the patient or with the family. Or the information might become the basis for a treatment decision such as whether to begin, continue, or stop a particular therapeutic regimen. We look at these issues and the concept of clinically significant decision levels in laboratory testing in Chapter 5.

All of these functions have traditionally belonged to the clinician. Others—collecting the specimen, performing the assay, and insuring the validity of the results—have been the hospital's or reference laboratory's responsibilities. When testing is moved to the physician's office or to the patient's home, however, the clinician must assume responsibility in these matters, as well. They are fully discussed in Part III, "The Analytical Practice of Office Testing."

As we've seen, laboratory testing in patient care involves the interaction of at least three factors: the clinician, the patient, and the analysis itself. The testing loop usually begins with the patient asking the clinician for help; it then follows the seven steps in Figure 1-1. As with any other chain, this one can be no stronger than its weakest link. Office testing can be only as sound as the clinician's understanding of the potential and the pitfalls in laboratory testing and of how to use the information generated, examples of which we discuss in Chapter 5.

With the return of the office laboratory, the physician must understand and control both the clinical (Part I) and the analytical (Part III) practice of the testing done there. This will help make it possible to produce the reliable, accurate, precise results that are necessary to meet today's standards of practice.

2

Selecting laboratory tests

After deciding that laboratory information is necessary to evaluate a patient's problem, the clinician takes the first step in the lab testing loop: selecting specific tests. This, of course, involves answering certain questions:

- Which test or tests will provide the information I need?
- In what sequence should I request these tests?
- When should I order them?
- How often should I order them?

Over the past few years, both the medical profession and the public at large have voiced concern about widespread misutilization of laboratory tests. Since clinicians initiate all laboratory test requests, they must bear the responsibility for this indictment if it is correct. The individual physician may not even be conscious of ordering too many or too few tests, of ordering tests too often or not frequently enough, of ordering the more expensive test when a cheaper test might do, or of subjecting the patient to greater risk of physical trauma when a readily available, less invasive, technique would be adequate.

Before trying to understand misuse of the laboratory, it is important first to address this question: "Why should laboratory tests be ordered at all?" There are, in fact, many situations in which no laboratory test is necessary. As examples, consider the evaluation of a patient with mild sunburn, one with possible ankle ligament strain, or one with a grief reaction. These situations all represent cases where laboratory testing would be quite superfluous to the clinician-patient interaction.

It must also be emphasized that laboratory testing represents only one type of clinical information. Others include the historical summary and results of the physical examination, radiologic examinations, and other special studies. Laboratory information supplements such data to help the clinician develop a diagnostic or medical management decision.

Given all these other possibilities, why should the physician order laboratory tests? There are four major reasons:

1. To detect (exclude) the possibility of a disease
2. To confirm the presence of a disease
3. To classify the type of disease
4. To monitor a patient's progress or response to therapy.

A MATTER OF CLASSIFICATION: THE PATIENT

The first three reasons relate to some aspect of having to classify patients—as healthy or ill, as having a particular problem or not, or as having greater risk of or predisposition to a particular disorder. In this section we consider three major factors involved in the classification process: patient, attribute, and clinical class. The patient is someone who relies on elements in the medical care-system for his or her health and well being and who, explicitly or implicitly, presents the physician with a clinical problem:

- Do I have some dread disease?
- Should I be concerned about my chest pain?
- Why does my stomach hurt?
- Is the medicine you gave me working?
- Has my cancer recurred?
- How long do you think I will live?
- Should I continue to take the drugs you prescribed for me?
- Should I see another specialist?
- Should I go to the hospital?

To answer such questions, the clinician must rely on two kinds of information. The first is general, a priori knowledge learned in medical school, by attending conferences, by talking to other physicians, or from past experience with other patients. Essentially, this kind of information includes knowledge of the relationship between clinical classes of patients and probable outcomes, depending upon the therapy invoked.

In addition, this kind of information encompasses the diagnostic specificity and sensitivity of clinical signs, clinical symptoms, physical findings, and laboratory tests. The sensitivity of a diagnostic procedure is the probability that individuals with a particular disease will have a positive result (a positive sign, symptom, physical finding, or test result). Diagnostic specificity is the probability that someone without the disease will have a negative result (sign, symptom, and so on). The last type of a priori knowledge is the prevalence (or incidence) of a particular disease and the population examined (nation, state, community, or group of patients with a particular constellation of symptoms).

The second kind of information available to the clinician is information unique to the patient being examined. It includes the chief complaint, the history of the present illness, a review of the physiologic systems, demographic information, physical examination findings, and, of course, laboratory test results.

ATTRIBUTES

It is in this context that we define the second factor—attribute. As used here, an attribute is a unit of patient-specific information that can be ascertained on the basis of history, physical examination, laboratory test results, or other special studies. Here are some examples: The patient smokes cigarettes, coughs up bloody mucus, has a serum sodium value of 115 mmol/L, or had x-ray studies showing opacity in the right thorax. Others might include a patient's response to therapy or the survival beyond a certain period of time.

A patient may also have many attributes that are waiting to be discovered. If the clinician doesn't look for them, critical information may be missed, leading to an error of omission. Conversely, seeking information about attributes that are unnecessary to the diagnostic process, particularly if it's costly or of high risk to the patient may lead to errors of commission or overuse of laboratory testing.

DEFINING AND SUPPORTING ATTRIBUTES

Table 2-1 illustrates defining and supporting attributes used to classify women as pregnant and not pregnant. The defining attribute is the birth of an infant; but it is obviously important to determine the probability of pregnancy before that event. When we don't have proof of the defining attribute, we must rely on ancillary information, or supporting attributes. Each of these, alone or in combination, could be used to estimate the probability that the patient is (or is not) a member of class A (pregnant). Obviously, with time, additional supporting attributes will make such a judgment 100% reliable.

In this simple example, one can see the relationships between clinical class, patient, and types of attributes. Most clinical decisions are based on the knowledge that a patient is a member of one or more clinical classes. In the situation described here, this judgment can be verified by observing the patient herself. In other cases, we may not have verification of a defining attribute.

Table 2-2 shows how patients can be classified into those suffering from an acute myocardial infarction (MI) and those who are not. In this discussion, only the patient who has died and had an autopsy demonstrating an MI can be classified with certainty (the defining attribute). If someone survives an episode presumed to be an MI, then verification would obviously not be 100% positive. Thus supporting attributes must frequently be used to make such a decision. The clinician usually classifies patients on the basis of a particular supporting attribute, such as an ECG abnormality. It is also relevant to question whether classification might be better based on an abnormal ECG or on the presence or absence of an elevated CK-MB value.

WHAT IS A CLINICAL CLASS?

Now for the third factor: A clinical class is defined here as a group of patients with one or more attributes in common. Patients can be placed in several actual or theoretical classes. They can, for example, be separated into male and female classes, into those with elevated and normal serum sodium values, and into those who will live to be 70 years or older and those who won't. The critical issue is to decide when such classification is clinically relevant, that is, when it will lead to selecting specific courses of therapy, give relevant prognostic information, or suggest the need for more clinical information.

The classification scheme has a number of steps. Some may involve making assumptions (as when the defining attribute is unknown), and others involve computations (Table 2-3).

TABLE 2-3

Steps in classification

1. Define the class explicitly and with assurance.
2. Remember that a patient is either a member of a class or not.
3. When you know the defining attribute (the one that explicitly characterizes a class), you can assign someone to that class with certainty.
4. When you do not know the defining attribute, you can determine only the probability that someone belongs to the class by considering supporting attributes.

CONSEQUENCES OF ASSIGNING PATIENTS TO A CLASS

Decisions to act are based partly on knowing (with varying degrees of assurance) that a patient belongs to a particular clinical class. Consequently, it is imperative to have as much information (supporting attributes) as possible to make such assignments.

- If a patient is definitely not a member of a clinical class, then the condition, by definition, is excluded.
- If the patient is definitely a member of a clinical class, the condition is confirmed.
- If there is uncertainty about whether or not a patient belongs to a clinical class, the condition cannot be excluded or confirmed. In such cases, laboratory measurements may be helpful to exclude, confirm, or detect the condition. This book, devoted to office laboratory medicine, will deal primarily with clinical problems for which laboratory tests may help classify patients with some degree of assurance. Obviously, for other clinical problems, information derived from the patient's history, the physical examination, x-ray, and other special studies may be of more assistance.

THE IDEAL LABORATORY TEST

The ideal test is one that discriminates between clinical classes with 100% assurance. One such test would be measure of sickle cell hemoglobin. The clinical problem is to distinguish patients with sickle cell trait from those without it. In this case, the defining attribute is the presence or absence of hemoglobin S as noted on the electrophoretogram. Classification is possible, even if no other tests are done, because the defining attribute is the same as the supporting one. As here, the ideal laboratory test should be relatively inexpensive, should not involve great risk to the patient, and should be 100% reliable analytically.

USING MATH IN MEDICINE

You may wonder at the mathematical turn we will be taking in this discussion. We offer this paragraph as a brief explanation. Feinstein[1] has defined mathematical symbolism as "a method of describing the relationship of things that people think about." He points out that clinicians may be startled to discover that they

Is the patient ill?

Class A: Ill patient = 1
Class B: Well patient = 0

Defining attribute: Independently confirmed state of health

Supporting attribute: BUN value

Note: All BUN values $\geq$ 28 mg/dL = 1
      All BUN values < 28 mg/dL = 0

---

think in mathematical sets at every stage of diagnosis, estimating prognosis, therapeutic decision making, and correlation of clinical laboratory data. In short, people use mathematic symbolism to think more clearly, and it is perhaps the best way to analyze the complicated reasoning processes inherent in diagnosis.

THE SINGLE TEST AS A DETECTOR OF DISEASE: BUN AS AN EXAMPLE

Let us examine two clinical classes: people who are ill and those who are well. We are not concerned with the defining attribute here, which is independent knowledge of the person's health; but with the supporting attribute, which is a laboratory test estimating the serum urea content, or blood urea nitrogen (BUN). Essentially, this asks whether the patient is ill (Table 2-4).

Quantitative information is often transformed into a binary (dual-valued) mode. In this example, the BUN is coded either 1 or 0, and the patient's state of health is also coded 1 or 0. If the patient is ill, the attribute is labeled as 1. If the patient is not ill or has a physiologic but nonpathologic condition such as dehydration, the attribute is coded as 0. The definitions of the classes, of the supporting attributes, and of the coding scheme are detailed in Table 2-4. Reorganizing this analysis in the form of a 2 x 2 table of classes and attributes is shown in Table 2-5. This gives four distinct possibilities:

- Ill patient and elevated BUN = true positive;
- Ill patient and normal BUN = false negative;
- Healthy patient and elevated BUN = false positive;
- Healthy patient and normal BUN = true negative.

Defining true and false test results.

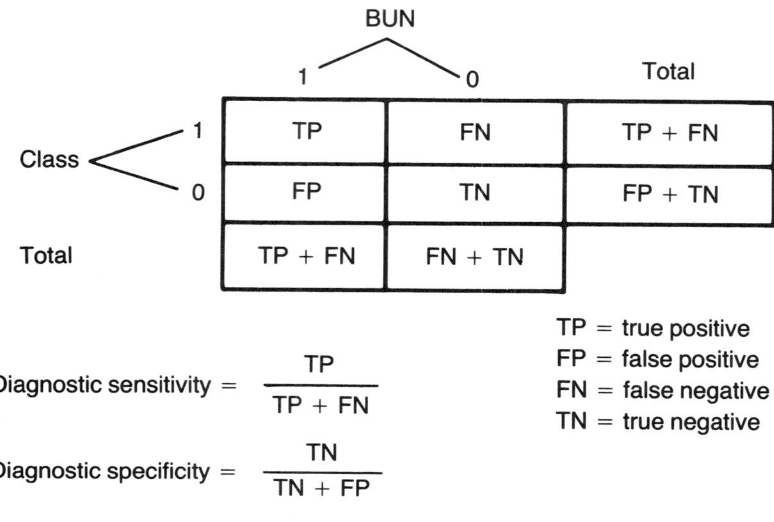

$$\text{Diagnostic sensitivity} = \frac{TP}{TP + FN}$$

$$\text{Diagnostic specificity} = \frac{TN}{TN + FP}$$

In addition, we can now define the terms diagnostic sensitivity and specificity. If a test is to be used as a screening test—to find all individuals with a serious, treatable disease—then it must have a very high (essentially 100%) sensitivity. If the BUN test is to be used to identify all sick patients, then by definition they will all have serum BUN greater than 28 mg/dL. If the single test is to be used to confirm illness, excluding any healthy people, then it should have a very high specificity. In this particular example, the BUN test was being proposed as a screening rather than a confirming test.

THE NEED FOR PREVALENCE INFORMATION

Determining diagnostic sensitivity and specificity is necessary but not sufficient to evaluate the use of supportive attributes when the group includes people from both classes. This is because there is a definable false-negative and false-positive rate. That is to say, not everyone with a positive test can be accurately classified as having the problem, and vice versa.

The predictive value of a positive test is an expression of the likelihood that someone with a positive test result actually be-

TABLE 2-6

How to determine predictive values

1. Define the clinical problem.
2. Define the supporting attribute.
3. Define the necessary probabilities:
   Prevalence of clinical classes
   Sensitivity
   Specificity
4. Determine predictive values with a two-by-two table.

---

longs to the class with the disorder—in our earlier example, that a patient with an elevated BUN value is actually ill. Conversely, the predictive value of a negative test is the likelihood that someone with a negative test is actually healthy. While the sensitivity and specificity are functions of the test and of the disorder being diagnosed, the predictive value is a function of the prevalence of the disorder in the population being tested.

Consequently, another fact is essential in our analysis of the patient classification problem: the prevalence of the various clinical classes in the population being studied. This is defined as the probability of a person's being in one class or the other. Prevalence information, essential to computing the predictive value of a supporting attribute, can be obtained from epidemiologic studies based on predefined criteria.

The credit for defining the predictive value model based on the notions of prevalence, diagnostic specificity, and diagnostic sensitivity should be given to Bayes[2] for his treatise written over 200 years ago. More recently, Galen and Gambino[3] popularized this model and applied it to evaluating the usefulness of clinical laboratory information in diagnostic and management processes.

The four steps used to determine the predictive values of a positive or negative test are outlined in Table 2-6. As noted there, the first step is defining the clinical problem: assigning patients to either the ill or healthy class of subjects is the example. The next step is defining the supporting attribute: The BUN determination with a value of greater than 28 mg/dL is a positive result and a value of less than 28 mg/dL is considered negative. The third step is defining the necessary probabilities: in this case, de-

---

Two-by-two table for 100,000 patients

BUN

		Positive	Negative	Total
	Ill	5,000	5,000	10,000
Class	Well	4,500	85,500	90,000
	Total	9,500	90,500	100,000

$$PV\,(+) = \frac{5,000}{9,5000} = 52.6\%$$

$$PV\,(-) = \frac{85,500}{90,500} = 94.5\%$$

---

termining these important prevalence values, which were determined by Martin and his co-workers[4]:

- the probability (prevalence) of finding a sick patient when the subject is chosen at random is 10%;
- the probability of finding a healthy subject under the same conditions is therefore 90%.
- the probability of finding a positive BUN result when the subject is ill is 50%, which is the test's sensitivity;
- the probability of finding a negative value when the patient is healthy is 95%; which is the test's specificity.

Having all this information, the next step is to determine the predictive value, either with a two-by-two table or the Bayes theorem. The table can be constructed with the information assuming a total population of 100,000 individuals (Table 2-7). From this, it can be seen that if a given subject has a positive test, there is a 52.6% probability (the predictive value of a positive test [PV +]) that the individual is ill. The predictive value of a negative test (PV −) is 94.5%.

Remember that sensitivity and specificity define the reliability of a test in a particular clinical situation; that is, the test's ability to distinguish diseased individuals from those who are not.

Sensitivity is a test's ability to give a positive result when a person truly has the disease; a test's specificity is its ability to give a negative result when the person is free of disease. Thus a test with no false-negative errors would be considered the most sensitive test, and a test with no false-positive errors would qualify as 100% specific for the disease under investigation.

CLINICAL APPLICATIONS OF SENSITIVITY, SPECIFICITY, AND PREDICTIVE VALUE

The concepts of sensitivity, specificity, and predictive value can have direct bearing on selecting tests to diagnose and manage clinical problems. There are circumstances, for example, when it is important to find all, or almost all, of the individuals with a particular problem. An example would be in screening for a disease with significant morbidity and mortality in which early treatment greatly improves the outcome. Finding everyone with the disorder can be done by subjecting high-risk individuals who have been identified by a highly sensitive, but less specific test to a second test of very high specificity to confirm the diagnosis. The next section will discuss such multiple testing strategies.

The efficient use of a test depends greatly on the composition of the population being tested and the prevalence of disease in that population. The predictive value of a positive CK test result, for example, depends on whether the patient is in the CCU to rule out MI, where the prevalence is 50%, or has been admitted for elective repair of an inguinal hernia and has had a routine admission chemistry profile. The possibility of MI in this patient is probably one in 1,000 admissions or less. Given these circumstances, a positive CK for the CCU patient has a predictive value of 90% while that of a positive CK for the asymptomatic surgery patient is 0.9% (Figure 2-1).

Another way of using prevalence information is to note that the test in the CCU raised the probability of MI from 50% to 90% while the probability of an MI in the surgery patient increased from 0.1% to 0.9%. Such testing is most helpful when uncertainty is greatest (when the probability is close to 50%); it is of less help when the probability is either very high or very low because it is unlikely that a positive test result will change the clinical management.

Except for screening tests, when the prevalence of a disorder in the population can be tested, the literature offers little

How changing prevalence affects the efficiency of CK testing to identify AMI patients

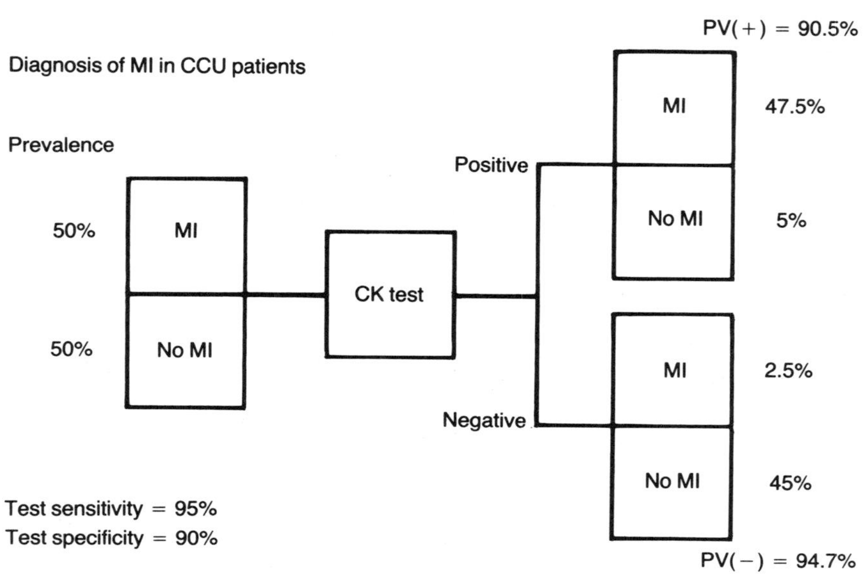

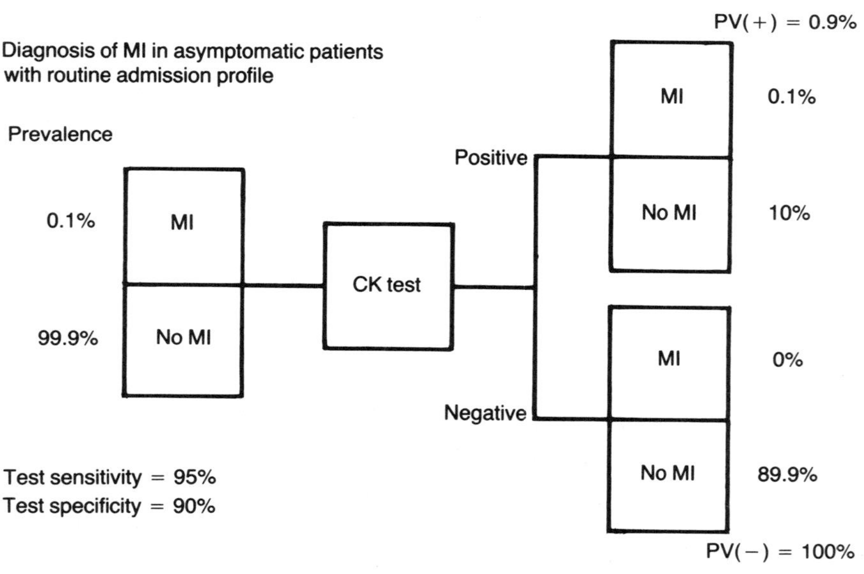

guidance in defining disease prevalence in a certain population. Clinicians, as part of their diagnostic skills, are in fact continually involved in assessing the likelihood of a problem in their own patients. The language most often used is descriptive rather than quantitative, but the physician is constantly making decisions about whether symptoms are potentially ominous and demand close follow-up or whether the danger is small, requiring less surveillance. As we've noted, a positive test probably won't change the clinical impression when another diagnosis is highly likely, but it will often be helpful in selecting a direction between two equally probable diagnoses.

MULTIPLE TESTING

As mentioned, a single test (or for that matter any diagnostic intervention) may not always be enough to differentiate the diagnoses under consideration. In such cases, multiple tests often facilitate the process. Ordering more than one test can be done at the same time—such as requesting both a total thyroxine and a T_3 uptake test to compute the free thyroxine index—or sequentially—such as ordering a serum albumin after noting a reduced serum calcium value.

A sophisticated mathematical approach called discriminant function analysis has been used to evaluate such simultaneous test ordering in given situations, but the clinician can usually evaluate two or more test results intuitively, without relying on such formulations. Today, of course, automated data processing gives us new opportunities to assess the value of multiple testing. Tests may also be selected and ordered sequentially on the basis of results of the initial diagnostic assessment or on the basis of laboratory information acquired during the evaluation. We'll discuss such testing strategies in Chapter 5, as we describe selected clinical problems. Other treatments of the structured approach, such as the use of clinical algorithms based on laboratory measurements, may be found in Lundberg's *Using the Clinical Laboratory in Medical Decision Making*.[5]

CHOOSING OFFICE TESTS: CLINICAL RELEVANCE AND PRACTICAL CONSIDERATIONS

The availability of timely test information—and of many tests never before found in the clinician's office—will certainly change the office practice of medicine in the coming years. Using these procedures, particularly those most helpful in deciding which patients require further care or evaluation, will mean that the clinician must become conversant with some of the clinical and technical issues related to the test itself.

Sedimentation rates are commonly used to screen for inflammation and occasionally to monitor the activity of established inflammation, as in systemic lupus erythematosus. For the latter, the Westergren sedimentation rate (or one of its satisfactory modifications) is a good test, with the sedimentation rate value continuing to increase with the progressively higher plasma concentrations of macromolecules associated with increased disease. The test is less sensitive, however, to the smaller increment in macromolecule concentration found with a less severe or focal inflammation (as in a patient with a focal pneumonia). For these cases, the Wintrobe sedimentation rate is more sensitive. Thus, the Wintrobe method would be more suitable for screening in the family practitioner's office and the Westergren in the rheumatologist's practice. The Wintrobe test is done with undiluted whole blood, and its results plateau when the inflammatory process is moderately severe; Westergren test results become progressively more abnormal.

Microbiology tests are also becoming increasingly available for the office practice. They must be used cautiously, however, and their diagnostic efficiency appreciated as well. For example, performing conventional microbiologic tests for gonorrhea—culture in the female and the urethral smear in the male—requires technical expertise in order to obtain a meaningful result. Moreover, even in the best of hands, the sensitivity of the reference method for diagnosing gonorrhea in women (identifying the organism in culture) is only 75% to 85% with a single specimen and 85% to 95% if two separately collected specimens are analyzed. Difficulty in isolating the organism is due to its fragility outside the biologic host and is related to how carefully the specimen was collected. Continued practice is necessary to identify the organism on urethral smears, particularly when it's in low concentration, and the quality of specimen collection is the foundation on which accurate diagnosis rests.

In considering alternative diagnostic approaches to this clinical problem, the clinician today has two options: an immunoassay to identify the organism from culture and a serologic test to detect antibodies to gonorrhea. An adaptation of the former may soon be available for a direct test on the specimen. In considering which of these tests to use in the office laboratory, the physician must try to make sure that the test produces the information it promises without ambiguity. In the case of gonorrhea, for example, the test for serum antibody is indeed sensitive, but it is not very specific for an active infection because the antibody may be the result of a past infection.

Coagulation tests are considered next. Standardization of these highly technical procedures is essential, but the necessary materials are expensive and not completely satisfactory. Thus the clinician is obliged to work closely with a reference laboratory, often in the hospital where these patients might be sent. In this way, results from the office laboratory should be comparable with those obtained in the hospital.

Clinical chemistry tests such as potassium, glucose, and uric acid should certainly facilitate the office management of hypertensive patients taking thiazide diuretics. It will be important for the clinician to realize that some precision may be sacrificed for the immediacy of the result. One procedure available for the office, for example, offers a potassium method in which the coefficient of variation (CV, see the glossary in Chapter 17) is 4% to 5% compared with less than 1% in methods used in a hospital-based laboratory. Thus the true potassium (95% confidence limits) will be between 5.4 and 6.6 mEq/L when the office test result is 6.0 mEq/L (the mean plus and minus twice the CV). When clinicians take these tests into the office, they will have to be aware of the level of precision of each assay and any common interfering substances (Table 3-4 in Chapter 3) inasmuch as these might change the interpretation of the result.

With some tests, the clinician will want to delve into issues the hospital laboratorian usually addresses. For example, current methods for measuring CK-MB use electrophoresis or column chromatography to separate the CK isozymes. The sensitivity and specificity of the two commonly used methods are quite different. There is no apparent problem when this test is applied to patients in the acute-care setting, but diagnostic problems do occur when the column chromatography test is applied to an unselected population to screen for AMI (Figure 2-2 compares the two tests). The high rate of false-positive results in an unselected population is potentially hazardous to their health. A positive

How different sensitivity and specificity affect the efficiency of CK-MB testing in identifying MI patients.

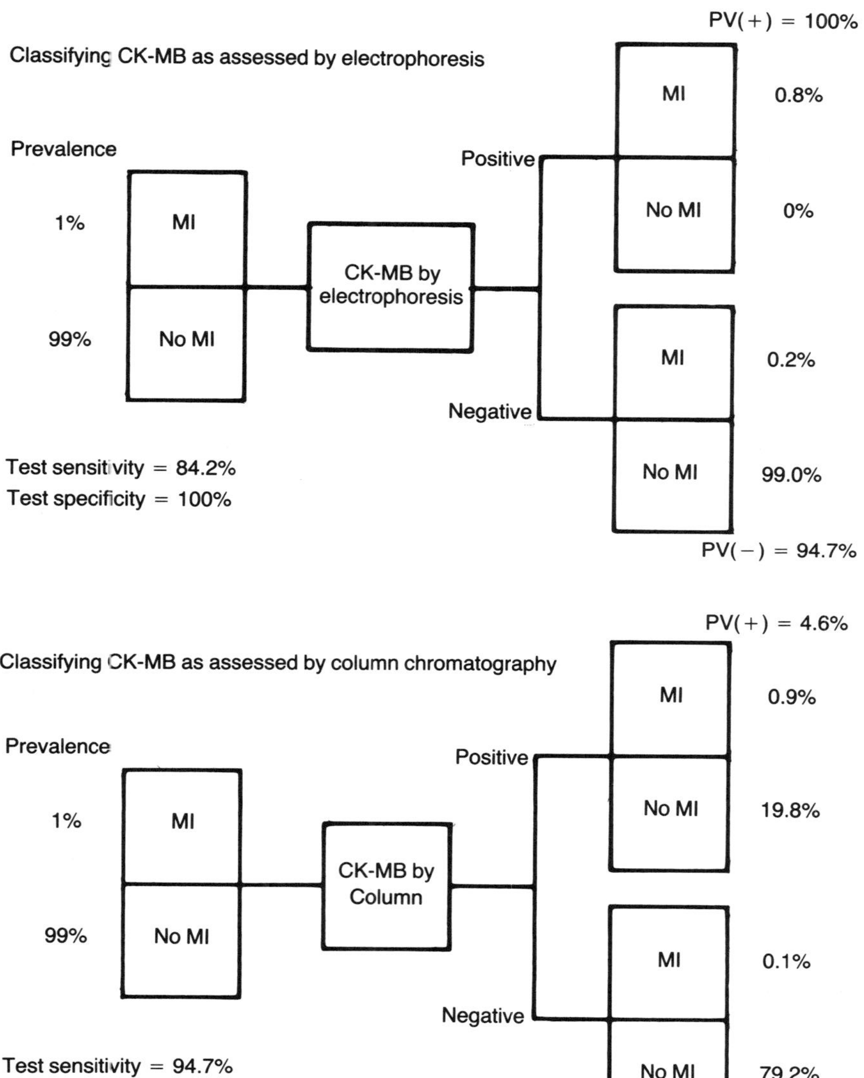

CK-MB test would prejudice the patient's ability to secure life insurance, for example.

The office laboratory can easily help diabetics who use capillary glucose monitoring to produce reliable results at home. Using specimens drawn in the office, the lab can compare its results with those the patient obtains and thus identify anyone having trouble with the analysis. Again, since the methodologies used by the patient and the office lab may be similar, it will be important for the physician to establish a relationship with a reference laboratory to ensure the accuracy of the determinations.

This common test is widely used and has been standardized so that a result from one laboratory should be comparable with that from another. The physician must make sure that the office laboratory is also producing comparable results. It is not enough to accept a manufacturer's assurance of comparable performance since the simplified equipment for this setting requires some site-dependent operator functions. We'll describe diabetic management more completely in Chapter 16.

As we discuss in Chapter 4, most testing systems are supplied with normal (reference) values for each test. It's most important for the office practitioner to validate the local application of these norms to the particular locale or practice. It is clear, for example, that hemoglobin norms developed for patients at sea level are inappropriate for Denver. It is similarly inappropriate to use uncritically the published norms for glucose and creatinine in a predominantly geriatric practice. The clinician should consult with local laboratorians for help with setting reference values.

A FINAL WORD

When you're approaching a decision about ordering a test, it is important to estimate the likelihood that a significant result would really add to the patient's management. This means considering three questions, as LaCombe suggests.[6]
- Will results of this test change the diagnosis, prognosis, or therapy?
- Will these results provide a better understanding of the patient's disease?
- What am I looking for and why? Would the patient benefit if I find it?

Misutilization of laboratory tests is not synonymous with overutilization; it also includes delayed or underutilization of appropriate testing. Failure to order a serum drug level when a patient is being evaluated for drug toxicity, failure to order a serum thyroxine test to evaluate someone who might be suffering from hypothyroidism, or failure to determine the antibiotic susceptibility of an organism in a patient with bacteremia are all serious errors of omission. Each clinical situation must be evaluated uniquely, so as to weigh the cost and benefit of ordering a test versus not ordering it in the diagnostic or management process.

REFERENCES

1. Feinstein AR: An analysis of diagnostic reasoning: 3. The construction of clinical algorithms. *Yale J Biol Med* 1974;47:5-32.

2. Bayes T: An essay toward solving a problem in the doctrine of chance. *Philos Trans R Soc* 1763;53:370.

3. Galen RS, Gambino SR: *Beyond Normality: The Predictive Value and Efficiency of Medical Diagnosis.* New York, John Wiley & Sons, 1975.

4. Martin HF, Gudzinowicz BJ, Fanger H: *Normal Values in Clinical Chemistry: A Guide to Statistical Analysis of Laboratory Data.* New York, Marcel Dekker, Inc, 1983.

5. Lundberg, GD: *Using the Clinical Laboratory in Medical Decision-Making.* Chicago, American Society of Clinical Pathologists, 1983.

6. La Combe MA: A six-point test ban treaty for house staff. *Resident Staff Physic* 1973;19:47-48.

3

Preparing the patient

After deciding to order one or more laboratory tests, the clinician takes the second step in the laboratory testing loop: preparing the patient. This includes telling the patient before collecting the specimen about any restrictions that may limit normal activities but are required for interpreting test results accurately.

The specimen may be collected as an emergency or as part of a plan. In the former setting (evaluating a patient complaining of acute chest pain, acute abdominal pain, or the acute onset of shortness of breath), there is relatively little opportunity for preparation. The priority is promptness, both in evaluating the patient and collecting the specimen.

In planned settings, such as an outpatient clinic, the situation is quite different. Testing can be scheduled far in advance, and the physician can talk to the patient about various preanalytical factors that influence test results. The patient should be instructed on how to control these factors by, for example, fasting or keeping a special diet, restricting ethanol ingestion or tobacco smoking, changing medication use or dosage, controlling changes in posture, and limiting exercise before the specimen collection.

The concentration of some analytes may vary with the time of day, the day of the month or of the menstrual cycle, or the seasons of the year. Such time-related factors are often governed by hormonal changes but may also relate to other, nonhormonal factors that are often more difficult to define. The latter may include such influences as exposure to sunlight, when a person

Preanalytical factors to consider

Diet or state of fasting	Caffeine	Exercise
Ethanol ingestion	Drugs	Time of collection
Tobacco smoking	Posture	

eats, and whether he has just finished a day of work or just gotten up in the morning (a marked posture change). An anomalous test result may seem to be caused by variation of some endogenous factor but may actually be related to an exogenous factor that was overlooked. Although it may be appropriate to restrict the specimen collection for some tests to a particular time (a serum cortisol in the early morning hours, for example), this is not necessary for most situations.

Now let us consider in turn various preanalytical factors that can affect laboratory values (Table 3-1).[1,2]

DIET

It is generally known that eating within a few hours before specimen collection may have an impact on selected laboratory results. A meal high in fat, for example, will increase serum triglycerides and alkaline phosphatase and cause various method-specific aberrations due to increased serum turbidity. This results in factitiously elevated or depressed values for analytes that are measured by light absorbance at a wavelength where lipid particles also absorb light. Since many of these interactions are instrument or method-specific, we will not discuss them further except to note that the interference caused by moderately hyperlipidemic serum may be overcome to a large extent by using adequate blanking (subtracting the initial absorbance from the final one) during the analysis or ultracentrifugation (the ordinary clinical centrifuge in the office laboratory is not adequate for this).

While the effects of postprandial laboratory testing are known, it is not as well appreciated that prolonged fasting (more than 24 hours) can also lead to unexpected laboratory findings. The typical consequences of a 48-hour fast on the results of a number of tests are listed in Figure 3-1. Notice that no significant

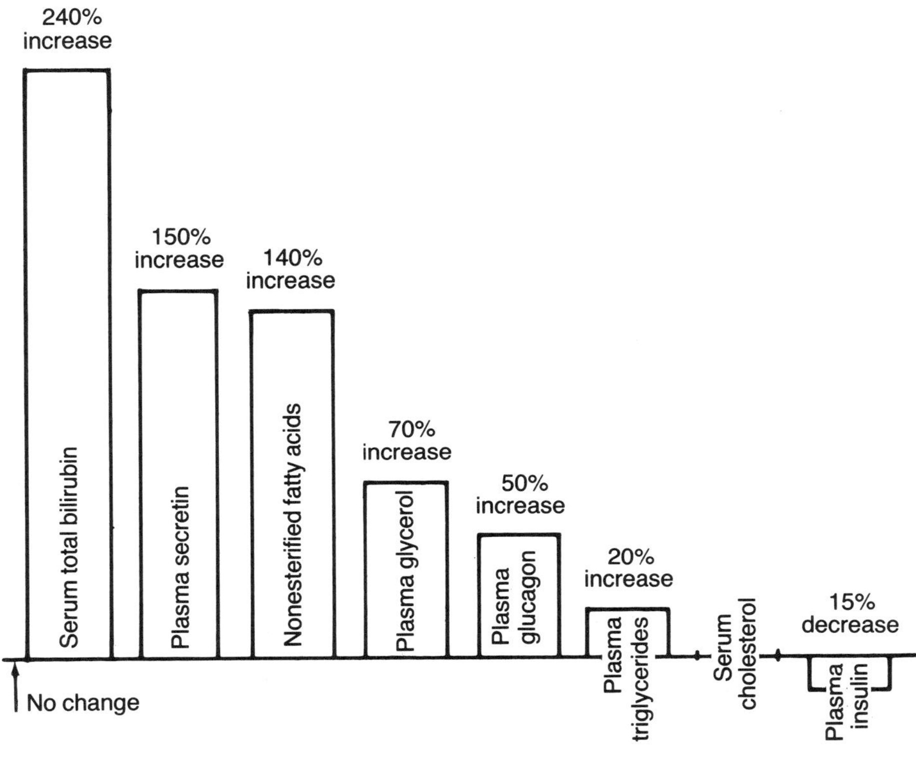

change occurs in the serum cholesterol concentration. It is also of note that plasma glucose levels can be expected to decrease to a mean value of 45 mg/dL in healthy adults who fast for more than 72 hours.

ETHANOL

Ethanol ingestion has both acute and long-term effects on various test results (Table 3-2). Short-term effects are usually the outcome of isolated episodes of drinking and are often seen in intoxicated patients with symptoms of hypoglycemia and metabolic acidosis in association with a high uric acid level. These patients may also have a number of other abnormal findings, including many of the serum enzyme activity tests. Fortunately,

Effects of ethanol ingestion

Acute (within 24 hours)

Plasma lactate	Increase
Serum urate	Increase
Serum bicarbonate	Decrease
Serum glucose	Decrease

Long-term (after two days)

GGT	Increase
HDL cholesterol	Increase
Serum triglycerides	Increase

most of these abnormalities are transitory and self-correcting within a day or two.

Long-term ethanol effects on test results are more likely to be found in chronic alcohol abusers. These patients frequently have abnormalities of several tests including an increased gamma-glutamyltransferase (GGT) as a result of acute ethanol ingestion or a chronic, alcohol-associated condition such as cirrhosis of the liver. If the former is the case, GGT values should decrease during hospitalization (assuming that the patient abstains from alcohol). The half-life of GGT is about six days; thus, a week after hospitalization, the GGT should be about half the value found at admission.

TOBACCO

Smoking has both acute and chronic sequelae that can influence laboratory test results. Acute effects include increases of plasma catecholamines and of serum cortisol, probably related to nicotine in tobacco. Changes in the concentration of these hormones in the blood can affect the total and the differential leukocyte counts—causing a decrease in eosinophils and an increase in neutrophils and monocytes. Other changes that may occur include elevations of plasma nonesterified fatty acids.

Chronic tobacco smoking can result in increases in blood hemoglobin values, the mean corpuscular volume (MCV), and the total WBC count. Heavy smokers who inhale may have carboxy-hemoglobin levels that account for as much 8% of the hemoglobin content of their blood (nonsmokers will have less than 1% of their hemoglobin as carboxyhemoglobin).

CAFFEINE

Most adults ingest at least 150 mg of caffeine daily, and we often find individuals getting three or four times that amount. The average cup of coffee—as well as certain black teas, colas, and other beverages—contains 100 to 150 mg of caffeine. It is metabolized by the liver, so patients with compromised hepatic function can have a prolonged caffeine half-life (normal: four hours). Caffeine ingestion is associated with increased plasma cortisol, catecholamines, and nonesterified fatty acids. Because of its effect on the concentration of the two stress hormones, caffeine may cause a falsely positive glucose tolerance test result.

It is difficult to assign precise numbers to test variations caused by caffeine because many variables can potentially maximize or minimize its impact. For example, the magnitude of the effect appears to be related to an intrinsic responsiveness to caffeine, whether the person is fasting or has recently eaten, and the time of day when the caffeine is ingested.

DRUGS

Drug interference with a laboratory test can be the consequence of a physiologic or pharmacologic effect in the patient or of a chemical effect on the analytic procedure.[3] Metabolites of some drugs can interfere in the measurement of certain analytes, particularly when drug concentration itself is being tested. Some drugs that interfere with commonly ordered laboratory tests are listed in Table 3-3.[4]

POSTURE

The influence of postural changes is particularly important when comparing results between inpatients and outpatients. In the office, for example, someone may have a serum albumin value of 3.8 g/dL. After that same patient has been hospitalized overnight, the albumin value may drop to 3.4 g/dL—solely as a result of being confined to bed. In general, the shift of body water asso-

Drugs that interfere with test results

Test	Drug	Effect	Mechanism
Albumin	Oral contraceptives	Decrease	Physiologic
Aspartate aminotransferase	Aspirin	Increase	Methodologic
	Isoniazid		
BUN	Furosemide	Increase	Physiologic
	Gentamycin		
Calcium	Hydrochlorothiazide	Increase	Physiologic
Creatinine	Amphotericin B	Increase	Physiologic
	Kanamycin		
	Salicylates		Methodologic
GGT	Oral contraceptives	Increase	Physiologic
	Phenobarbital		
	Phenytoin		
Glucose	Furosemide	Increase	Physiologic
	Hydrochlorothiazide		
Potassium	Furosemide	Decrease	Physiologic
	Hydrochlorothiazide		
	Spironolactone	Increase	
Prothrombin time	Warfarin	Increase	Physiologic
Serum thyroxine	Oral contraceptives	Increase	Physiologic
	Phenytoin	Decrease	
Sodium	Corticosteroids	Increase	Physiologic
	Hydrochlorothiazide	Decrease	
Uric acid	Allopurinol	Decrease	Physiologic
	Aspirin		
	Probenicid		
Urine color	Nitrofurantoin	Rust to yellow-brown	Methodologic
	Phenazopyridine	Orange-brown	

ciated with a healthy subject's standing up will result in an 8% to 10% increase in total serum protein concentration. The increment may be even greater in individuals with an excessive amount of fluid retention, as from congestive heart failure, for example.

When a person goes from a supine to an upright position, water and filterable substances travel from the intravascular to the interstitial fluid space. As a result, nonfilterable substances, such as proteins and cellular elements and the compounds associated with them, increase in concentration. Serum albumin levels, for example, increase when an individual changes from a supine to a standing posture. Since a substantial fraction of circulating calcium is bound to albumin, increases can also be expected in the serum calcium. Serum cholesterol, triglycerides, and bilirubin tend to follow the same pattern, since they are also bound to proteins. The serum concentration of drugs that are bound to serum proteins can also be expected to rise with this change in posture. Cellular elements in the blood that increase with standing up include hematocrit and the hemoglobin concentration because of the change in the disposition of the extracellular fluid volume.

EXERCISE

Exercise can have short- and long-term effects on various laboratory results. In a physician's office practice, the short-term effects are usually of minor significance, although they may be of interest to sports medicine specialists. These include changes in blood lactate, glucose, and hormone levels. The intermediate effects (one to two days after exercise) can often be the source of unexpected results. Exercise results in increased serum activity of certain enzymes usually found in muscle: creatine kinase (CK), aspartate aminotransferase (AST, SGOT), and lactate dehydrogenase (LD, LDH). Ten hours after exercise, it is not uncommon for the CK value to be twice the baseline levels and AST and LD values to be 50% above baseline.

Increased serum enzyme activity after exercise is related to several factors—vigor of the exercise, training of the participants, and timing of the specimen collection. The more strenuous the exercise and the more out of shape the subject, the higher the enzyme levels. Levels reach a peak in specimens collected five to 15 hours after the start of exercise.

THE TIME OF SPECIMEN COLLECTION

The following questions are related to the specimen collection time:

- Should blood be collected at a set time of day or anytime?
- Should a woman's blood or urine be collected at a particular day relative to the onset of menstruation?

Day-to-day variation in healthy people

Analyte (serum)	Coefficient of variation (%)
Electrolytes	
Sodium	0.7
Magnesium	1.3
Calcium	1.7
Chloride	2.1
Potassium	4.3
Phosphate	5.8
Metabolites	
Creatinine	4.3
Cholesterol	5.3
Glucose	5.6
Urate	7.3
BUN	12.3
Bilirubin	22.0
Triglycerides	25.0
Iron	26.6
Enzymes	
Gamma-glutamyltransferase	3.9
Alkaline phosphatase	4.8
Acid phosphatase	9.9
Lactate dehydrogenase	12.1
Aspartate aminotransferase (SGOT)	24.2
Creatine kinase	25.7
Alanine aminotransferase (SGPT)	26.4
Proteins	
Transferrin	2.5
IgG	2.7
Albumin	2.8
Total protein	2.9
IgM	3.1
IgA	3.5
Complement C3	3.8
Complement C4	5.9
Haptoglobin	8.8

- When is a change in a laboratory result related to disease, and when to nondisease sources of variation?

The specimen collection time as an intrinsic, nondisease source of variation can be separated into within-day and day-to-day variations. The former are those changes occurring within a 24-hour period of time, and they are usually most significant for hormone-related tests. The classic example is the ACTH-cortisol cycle. The peak ACTH value usually occurs during sleep, in the very early morning hours (about 4 AM); it is followed by the peak cortisol value about two hours later (between 6 and 8 AM). During the course of a day, both ACTH and cortisol dip to a third or a half their peak value. Sleep is also associated with increases in plasma growth hormone, gonadotropin, and other anterior pituitary hormone concentrations in the blood.

Another significant within-day change is variation in serum iron concentration, which peaks during the morning hours. The concentration of transferrin (the major iron-binding protein) does not vary significantly as a function of time of day, however. Most other analytes that have within-day changes do so unpredictably; the variations are random rather than systematic.

For most analytes, day-to-day variations are greater than within-day changes. Most of them are random, not varying because of menstrual cycle or of season, for example. Day-to-day variation is best characterized in terms of its intrinsic variance (expressed as the standard deviation [SD] or scatter). A unitless measure of percentage, the coefficient of variation (CV), can be derived by dividing the SD by the average value for the particular analyte. The concentration of serum electrolytes (sodium and potassium) varies less than 5% from day to day, for example. This is understandable since maintaining a tightly controlled electrolyte concentration in the blood is essential for the homeostatic balance. On the other hand, some serum enzymes vary up to 20% from day to day, although alkaline phosphatase (ALP) and GGT changes are usually limited to about 5%. The expected physiologic day-to-day variation of commonly ordered analytes in healthy subjects is shown in Table 3-4.[5]

It is well appreciated that the concentration of hormones controlling the menstrual cycle vary at different times during that cycle. When testing to assess menstrual irregularity, hirsutism, or infertility requires hormonal evaluation, it is critical for the clinician to realize that different reference values are appropriate during the cycle's different phases. This can be a particularly difficult problem in assessing a patient with oligomenorrhea or amenorrhea who has a high luteinizing hormone (LH) concentration in the blood; one cannot be sure whether this is the result of ovulation or a result of ovarian failure. In such cases, repeated measurements can clarify the situation since the ovulatory surge of LH is transient while the increased LH concentration as a result of ovarian failure is stable.

OTHER FACTORS

Prolonged tourniquet application can cause a modest increase in the concentration of nonfilterable blood substances. For example, total serum protein will be 3% to 4% higher when a tourniquet is left in place for three minutes instead of one minute before phlebotomy. Serum catecholamines also rise when a tourniquet is applied, but this is more a result of the patient's feelings of stress at having blood drawn than an effect of the physical application of the tourniquet.

It is difficult to evaluate the effect of stress on laboratory tests, but the increase in plasma catecholamines does trigger an increase in the concentration of plasma free fatty acids. Anxiety resulting in hyperventilation before venipuncture can lead to disturbances in measured acid-base balance—an increase in the blood pH due to a decreased partial pressure of carbon dioxide. Acute stress-induced plasma catecholamine increases can also cause a rise in total WBC count as a result of mobilizing the white cells in the marginating pool.

COLLECTING SPECIMENS FOR URINALYSIS

The quality of the information derived from urinalysis is highly correlated with the quality of the specimen. To minimize ambiguous results as a result of the specimen being contaminated with material from closely associated anatomic areas, most laboratorians recommend the collection of a clean voided midstream specimen for bacteriologic, chemical, and microscopic analysis. The recommended collection procedure will, of necessity, be different for men and women; special pediatric urine collectors of clear pliable polyethylene are available for infants.[6]

For women. The patient should straddle the toilet bowl and, with one hand, separate the vaginal labia. With the other hand, using sterile, soapy cotton balls, she should clean each side of the urinary meatus and then clean the urethral meatus itself. She should then rinse the cleansed area with sterile, water-saturated cotton balls and forcibly void, allowing the initial stream to go into the toilet. While still holding the labia apart, she should collect the subsequent stream in a clean container (sterile if it's for bacteriologic analysis).

For men. The patient should adequately expose the glans and clean it thoroughly using sterile, soapy cotton balls. In an uncircumcised man, it is important for him to retract the foreskin to avoid contamination from debris under the foreskin. After drying the glans with a sterile cotton ball, he should void, letting the initial stream fall into the toilet and then collecting the balance in a clean container.

IMPLICATIONS AND PRACTICAL INSTRUCTIONS

What should you take away from this chapter? First, that it may be important for you to instruct patients on various restrictions regarding diet, physical exercise, smoking, and drinking before collecting specimens for laboratory testing. Second, you should be aware of drugs the patient may be taking. It is occasionally critical to delay antibiotic therapy until after obtaining specimens for microbiologic analysis. Third, you should be aware of the effects of posture and tourniquet application on the results of certain laboratory tests.

In all cases, of course, the effects discussed in this chapter are most significant when the reference range is very narrow for a group of healthy subjects or when a subject is being monitored over time. In the latter case, variation in preparing the subject with its consequent variation of test results may obscure significant trends in the disease course.

For certain tests, explicit instructions—such as specifying a minimum amount of dietary carbohydrates for the three days before a glucose tolerance test—are given because the preparation is essential for unambiguous interpretation of the results. In certain clinical settings, other conditions may also affect laboratory measurements; examples include the effects of surgery, of hemodialysis, of parenteral nutrition, and of other disease unrelated to the problem being investigated. Since the clinician cannot manipulate these factors, we have not discussed them here. Nonetheless, when interpreting laboratory measurements, you should be aware that various therapeutic maneuvers, in addition to drugs, can cause profound changes in laboratory measurements. Occasionally, such effects may be so great that evaluating them becomes one more problem added to the list on the patient's chart.

REFERENCES

1. Statland BE, Winkel P: Effects of preanalytical factors on the intraindividual variation of analytes in the blood of healthy subjects. Consideration of preparation of the subject and time of venipuncture. *CRC Crit Rev Clin Lab Sci* 1977;8:105-144.

2. Statland BE: Nondisease sources of variation. *Diagnostic Medicine* 1984;July/August:60-64.

3. Young DS, Pestaner LC, Gibberman V: Effects of drugs on clinical laboratory tests. *Clin Chem* 1975;21:1D-432D.

4. Moskowitz MA, Osband ME: *The Complete Book of Medical Tests. A Lifetime Guide for You and Your Family.* New York, W W Norton & Co, 1984.

5. Winkel P, Statland BE: Using the subject as his own reference in assessing day-to-day changes of laboratory test results. *Contemp Top Clin Anal Chem* 1977;1:287-317.

6. Bradley M, Schumann GB: Examination of urine, in Henry JB (ed), *Clinical Diagnosis and Management by Laboratory Methods,* ed 17. Philadelphia, WB Saunders, 1984, pp 382-384.

4

Interpreting the results

Interpreting laboratory information is an intellectual way station on the road to definitive action. Indeed, laboratory results have true clinical relevance only after test values have been interpreted and some action has been taken to deal with the patient's problem.

The first step in interpretation is to compare the result with other information—either with values derived from other subjects (group-specific reference values) or from the patient (subject-specific values). In the latter case, we are looking at the effects of time on analyte concentrations (a time-series analysis).

NORMAL OR REFERENCE VALUES?

Until recently, most laboratorians were content to use the term "normal values." But this raises the question of defining just what normal means. Laboratorians generally use it to signify the middle 95% of values derived from a healthy population; most practicing clinicians, on the other hand, use the word to distinguish health from disease.

Largely because of such confusion, most laboratorians have come to prefer the term "reference values," which Grasbeck and Saris introduced in 1969.[1] Whenever we use reference values in this book, we will try to be explicit about the reference population and how the values have been derived.

ESTABLISHING GROUP-SPECIFIC REFERENCE VALUES

The steps used to establish reference values in a healthy population are listed in Table 4-1, and we'll discuss them in turn.

Step one: Defining health

A healthy individual might be described as someone with normal ambulatory function, a sense of well-being, no evidence of chronic disease, no recent illness, and no symptoms or signs of disease. But if we included the criterion of the absence of all signs of disease—including any abnormal laboratory measurements—it may be impossible to find even one healthy person in a hundred using the laboratory definition of normality.

Using that approach, reference (normal) values are defined here as the central 95% of the healthy population tested. They exclude, by definition, 5% of this population as having "abnormal" results for any single test. When more than one test is performed on a subject, the probability of finding an abnormal result in a "healthy" individual increases as a function of the number of tests ordered (Table 4-2). This theoretical presentation shows that nearly two thirds of healthy individuals subjected to a 20-test panel would have at least one "abnormal" result!

But if we say that abnormal laboratory results are not a basis for excluding people from the reference group, we must face the issue of our inability to always detect disease. For one thing, we can easily exclude people with a history or obvious symptoms or signs of illness. Those with subclinical or chronic disease may not have symptoms at the time they are used as part of the reference group, however. Someone with an occult neoplasm, for example, would probably be accepted in the presumably healthy volunteer group used to determine reference values. Thus, another approach to the definition of good health may be to establish it prospectively. For example, we could use survival time following specimen collection to establish reference values in a geriatric population.

In spite of such concerns, however, most laboratories continue to produce reference values for their population of so-called healthy individuals. And in practice, the values serve their purposes well.

Step two: Selecting a random subset population

It is important to be aware of the effect of such demographic factors as the age, sex, and race of the subject and, in women, whether they are pregnant.

Age. Pediatric reference values are often quite different from adult values, and for some analytes, they can vary with the age of the child as well. For example, newborns through the first week of life will have greatly elevated serum bilirubin levels and mildly increased serum gamma-glutamyltransferase (GGT), growth hormone, fetal hemoglobin, alpha-fetoprotein, and BUN values; they will have decreased serum carotene, ceruloplasmin, haptoglobin, and cholesterol values. In addition, healthy newborns will have dramatic increases in total WBC count and very low concentrations of IgM and IgA immunoglobulins in their plasma. These neonatal reference values can obviously be very important when evaluating the possibility of an infectious or an inherited disease.

TABLE 4-2

The probability of finding an abnormal result

Number of tests	Expected frequency (%) of one or more
"abnormal" results	
1	5
2	10
4	19
6	26
10	40
15	54
20	64

Compared with adult values, the pediatric subject before puberty generally has higher serum alkaline phosphatase (ALP), inorganic phosphate, and lactate dehydrogenase (LD, LDH) values, but significantly lower cholesterol, creatinine, serum uric acid, and total protein.

Menopausal women have higher reference values for ALP, cholesterol, inorganic phosphate, and uric acid than do younger women. And in both men and women older than 70, total protein values decrease, while ALP, cholesterol, creatinine, glucose, and BUN values increase.

Sex. Compared with women in the same age groups, men have higher reference values for BUN, creatinine, and serum uric acid before middle age (fifth or sixth decade). They also have higher reference values for calcium, serum lipids (triglycerides and cholesterol), and sodium. These sex differences in laboratory norms are probably related to differences in muscle mass and hormone balance.

Race. Oriental adults have lower serum cholesterol values but higher serum uric acid values than either white or black adults do. In general, blacks have higher—as much as 20% to 30%—serum creatine kinase (CK) and immunoglobulins, including IgA, IgG, and IgM, than whites.

Pregnancy. A number of dramatic changes occur in the blood chemistry of a pregnant woman when compared with the levels found in age-matched, nonpregnant women. Both the procoagulant and fibrinolytic factors are higher, and a pregnant woman's ALP values increase as a result of placental ALP isoenzyme in her serum. She also has higher aspartate aminotransferase (AST, SGOT), LD, serum lipid (cholesterol and triglycerides), and serum uric acid values. She has lower mean values of serum albumin, BUN, calcium, glucose, and total protein.

Step three: Obtaining and assaying the specimens

The fundamental assumption in a reference value study is that the population-derived values will be comparable to values of healthy patients found in the physician's practice. If reference values are being developed for an ambulatory-care setting, reference values should be derived from people who are upright, not supine. Test methodology should be the same for the reference and the practice groups.

Another important point is that reference value specimens should not be processed in one batch, just as specimens in the practice setting would not be batched. Processing in a single batch would also reduce the overall variation by eliminating the day-to-day component of analytical variance. To repeat, the key point is that comparability between the reference value group and the clinical practice is essential for appropriately interpreting a patient's test results.

Step four: Analyzing the data statistically

The data collected from the reference value study can be analyzed using various statistical approaches. The first, a parametric analysis of the untransformed (raw) data, is ideal and the most direct. If it appears that this method is not satisfactory—if the data are not conforming to a normal, Gaussian distribution, for example—the same kind of approach can be used on transformed data. If neither of these statistical approaches is satisfactory or appropriate, then a nonparametric approach can be used.

PARAMETRIC APPROACH USING RAW DATA

This method is based on the assumption that results from the reference value study will follow a symmetrical, bell-shaped Gaussian distribution and be essentially infinite in its spread. Obviously, this last characteristic is never represented with real, finite data. The Gaussian distribution is such that the interval enclosed by the mean minus two standard deviations (SD) and the mean plus two SD encompasses approximately 95% of the data points. Thus the reference interval is generally defined as the range of values representing 95% of the normal, healthy subjects used in the study.

PARAMETRIC APPROACH USING TRANSFORMED DATA

When the preceding method does not give a reasonable or usable reference range, it may be helpful to use transformed data. A common way to transform raw data is to compute the logarithm of each value and then analyze the new values with the same statistical analysis detailed earlier. Other approaches include computing the logarithm of each data point plus a constant, or determining the square root of each data point. Transformed values are always used to determine the reference intervals of certain analytes—serum enzymes, bilirubin, and total lipids. Thus serum triglyceride values that are collected as part of a reference value study may not result in a perfect Gaussian distribution, but the approximation is adequate for clinical use.

NONPARAMETRIC APPROACH

The values for some analytes do not lend themselves to analysis by conventional statistical methods with either raw or transformed data. In such cases, an alternative, nonparametric approach can be used. This does not depend on any preconceived notion as to what the distribution of the values actually is. Instead, the middle 95% is arbitrarily defined as the reference range. Then the highest 2.5% and the lowest 2.5% of the values are excluded, and the reference range becomes the middle 95% interval of what remains.

ESTABLISHING PATIENT-SPECIFIC
REFERENCE VALUES

The rationale for using patient-specific intervals is based on the fact that individual values vary less than group reference values do.[2] To put this in another light, patient-specific values are most helpful when the intra-individual variation is much less than the group variation. The ratio of the individual's variation to the group's variation for many analytes has, in fact, been used to suggest that subject-specific reference values provide better information for managing a particular patient than do group-specific values.

Intra-individual variation may be of two kinds: within-day circadian variation and day-to-day variation. Assuming that it's possible to obtain specimens at the same time every day, we need to be concerned only with the latter. Among the analytes with relatively small intra-individual, day-to-day variation compared with inter-individual variation, are ALP, GGT, specific serum proteins, and certain hematologic parameters.

Subject-specific reference values can be used to monitor patients for recurrence of a malignancy, to evaluate the effect of

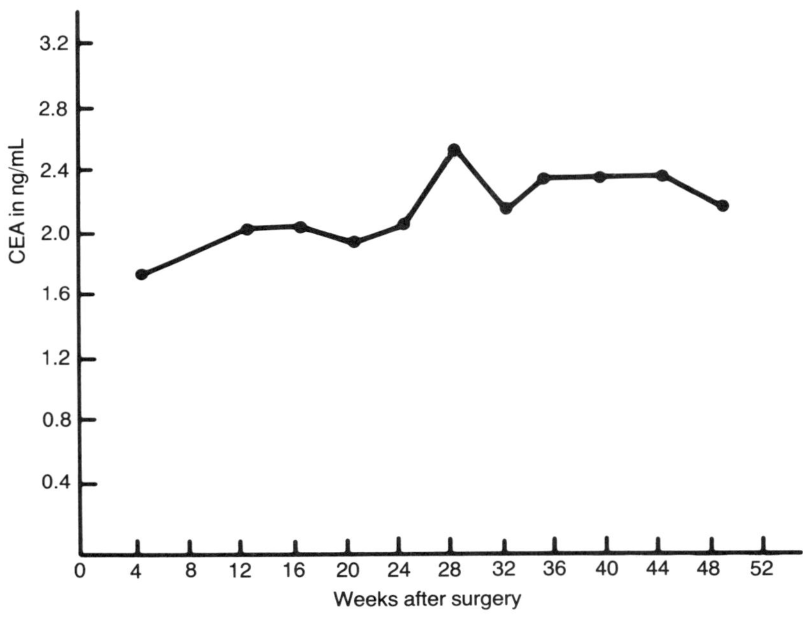

CEA values in a patient with breast cancer who had no known recurrence for 18 months after the last value shown

therapy in hyperlipoproteinemia, or to find out whether a transplanted organ is being rejected. In fact, using laboratory information to monitor the progression of any health problem or a patient's response to therapy of necessity involves the use of subject-specific reference values.

Carcinoembryonic antigen (CEA) values from a patient with breast cancer who had no tumor recurrence for 18 months after the last value are shown in Figure 4-1. This contrasts markedly with CEA values in a patient whose recurrence was noted soon after the last specimen was obtained (Figure 4-2). Using subject-specific CEA reference values made it possible to detect recurrence in the latter patient much earlier than if a fixed threshold cutoff value had been used.[3,4]

CEA values in a patient whose tumor recurrence was noted shortly after the last value shown

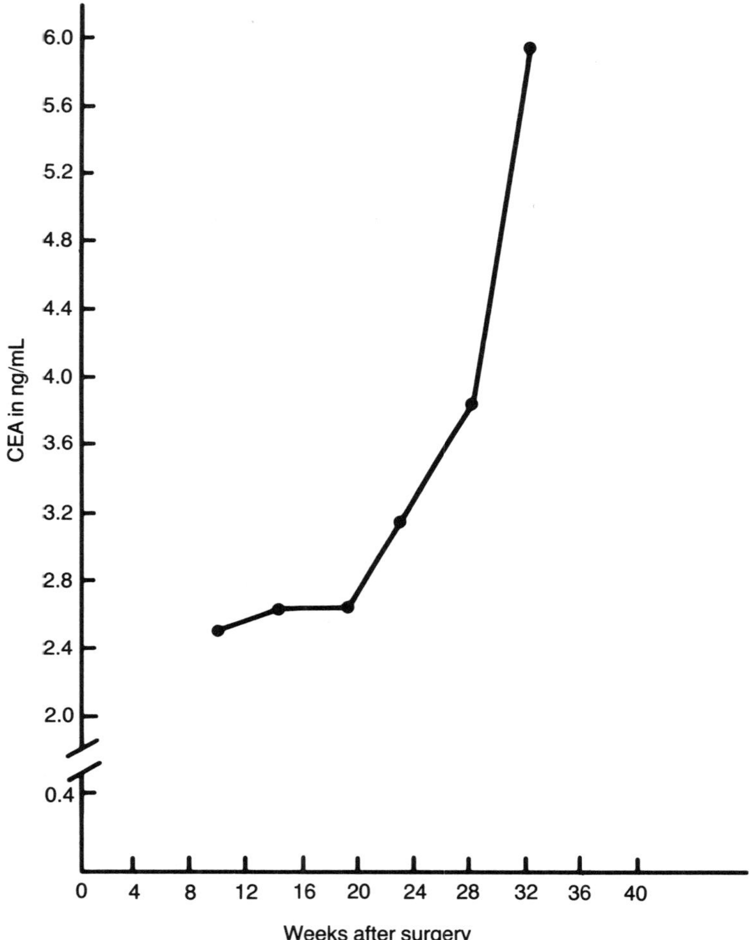

THE SIGNIFICANCE OF THE REFERENCE INTERVAL

When a patient value lies outside reference limits, we can make only a general inference: The patient is not a member of the group from which the sample population was selected. And in such a case, one of the following statements is true:

- The patient is sick.
- The patient is well, but is a statistical outlier.
- The patient is well, but is demographically different from the reference population.
- The patient is well, but the specimen was prepared differently from those of the reference population.
- The patient is well, but engaged in certain activities before the specimen was collected that caused lab values to be outside the reference limits.
- Analytical variance caused a spurious test result.

It's unfortunate that the clinician relies exclusively on a reference interval to answer the question, "Is the patient ill?" In fact, a person could be ill, but have a value for a particular analyte within the reference interval. Conversely, the patient could be well but have a value outside the reference range. The reason reference values can be somewhat misleading is that the alternative question is not asked: "What should we conclude when the value is outside the reference limit?" This problem and its solution will be discussed in the following chapter.

REFERENCES

1. Gräsbeck R, Saris NE: Establishing the use of normal values. *Scand J Clin Lab Invest* 1969;24(Suppl 110):62-65.

2. Harris EK: Effects of intra- and interindividual variation on the appropriate use of normal ranges. *Clin Chem* 1974;20:1535-1542.

3. Winkel P, Statland BE: Using the subject as his own reference in assessing day-to-day changes of laboratory test results. *Contemp Top Clin Anal Chem* 1977;1:287-317.

4. Winkel P, Bentzon MW, Statland BE, et al: Predicting recurrence in patients with breast cancer from cumulative laboratory results: A new technique for the application of time series analysis. *Clin Chem* 1982;28:2057-2067.

5

Acting on laboratory results

The real value of a laboratory measurement lies in its ability to affect patient management. If the outcome of a test will have no effect, it should probably not be performed. Testing can lead to three possible actions:

- Changing a patient's therapeutic regimen.
- Ordering additional diagnostic tests.
- Sharing prognostic information with the patient or the family.

CLINICAL DECISION-MAKING BASED ON LABORATORY RESULTS

The first step in this process is selecting the laboratory test. The next is deciding whether the test result exceeds predetermined limits (the discriminant values). If it does, one action will be taken; if it does not, another action will be called for (Figure 5-1). Such decision levels are required for every result in the decision-making process.[1] Examples of decision levels and subsequent actions include the following:

- Ordering a serum parathyroid hormone test (PTH) when a serum calcium value exceeds 11.0 mg/dL.
- Recommending an exchange transfusion when a newborn's serum bilirubin value exceeds 20 mg/dL.

Decision analysis based on a laboratory value

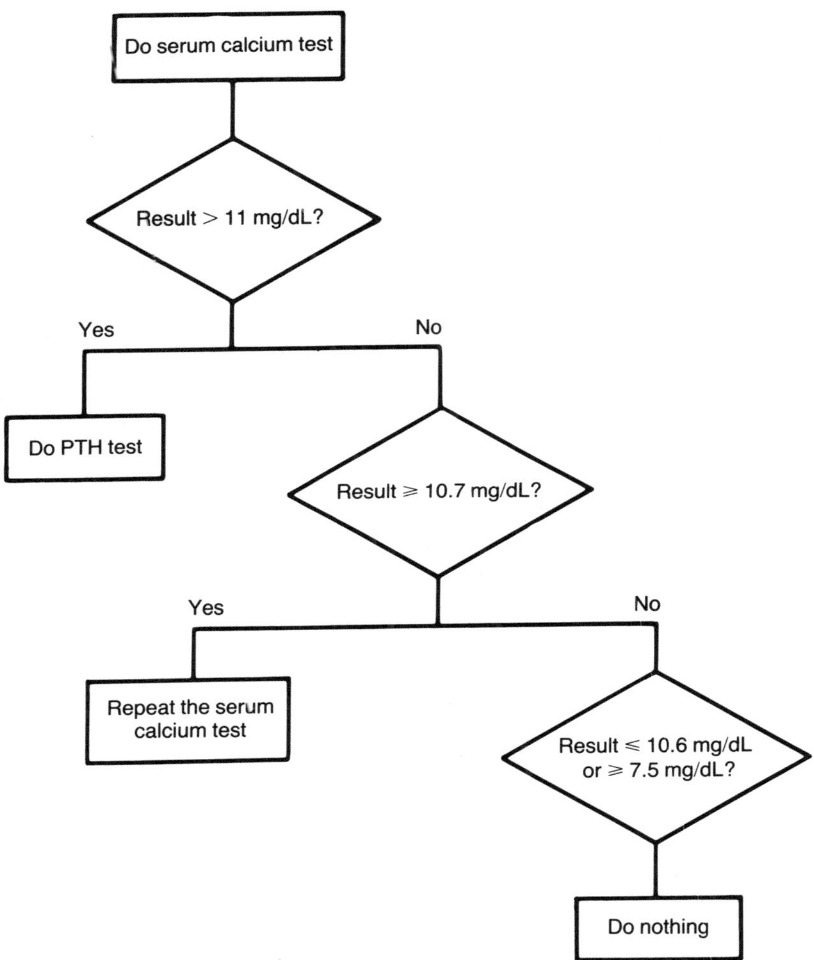

In this example, two courses of action are determined by comparing the value of a lab result with a predefined decision level.

- Submitting a blood specimen for a differential when the total WBC exceeds 12,000.
- Reducing the digoxin dosage in a patient with signs of toxicity when the serum digoxin concentration exceeds 1.6 ng/mL.

These examples describe the action taken for each clinical decision level. And some of them show how inappropriate it can be for clinicians to rely solely on reference values to make their management decisions. As we have said, it is not adequate simply to determine whether the result is outside a reference interval. As the product of a statistical stratification of an otherwise healthy population, reference values are no help in some of these situations.

In fact, most tests used in making clinical decisions do not have a single, unambiguous boundary between two alternative courses. More often, a sound decision requires at least two discriminant (threshold) values. The first describes the boundary that clearly identifies one class (and dictates one of the actions) while the second identifies the second class with its different course of action.

The example in Figure 5-2 shows two decision levels, DL_1 and DL_2. When the value of the test result exceeds DL_2, the patient almost certainly suffers from disease B, and appropriate therapy should be initiated. When the test value is less than DL_1, the subject is almost certainly healthy and needs no treatment. When the value lies between DL_1 and DL_2, however, we cannot confidently classify the subject as healthy or diseased, and we may want to order more tests.

How do decision levels DL_1 and DL_2 compare with the reference value limits for the test in question? The lower reference limit is obviously far from either decision level, but the upper reference limit is close to, but not identical with, the limit of the higher discriminant value, DL_2.

The balance of this chapter deals with a series of common clinical problems where laboratory tests may help. Throughout these examples, we discuss certain cutoff points—or decision levels—for specific actions. In each case, based upon the patient, the therapy available, and other local considerations, the clinician may use one or more of the proposed discriminant values in selecting laboratory tests to help make clinical decisions. The process of making the clinical decision must take into consideration

Theoretical distribution of subjects for a laboratory measurement

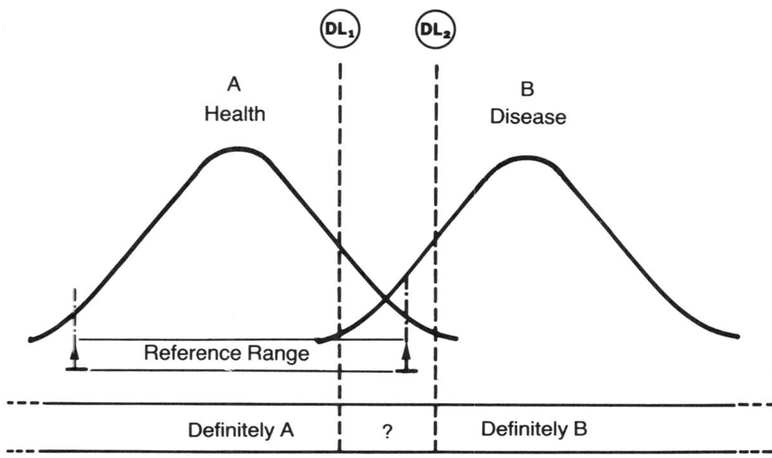

Source: Statland BE: *Clinical Decision Levels for Lab Tests*. Oradell NJ, Medical Economics Books, 1983, p 10.

the cost (including any risk) and benefit of intervening (initiating therapy, for example) compared with the cost and benefit of doing nothing.

Formal decision analysis involves considering the consequences of various interventions used to diagnose or manage a particular problem (such as acute abdominal pain) in a defined population (young women in the reproductive age range, for example). For each action, the probability of various outcomes such as recovery, continued morbidity, or death are calculated as are a positive or negative risk value and cost estimates for each intervention or outcome. The operating characteristics of various diagnostic tools can also be factored into the cost-benefit analysis, taking into consideration the risk and cost of false positives and false negatives (Chapter 2), which are implicit in the use of imperfect testing tools. With such an approach, it is possible to estimate, quantitatively and formally, the cost and benefit of each of many interventions for diagnosing or managing a particular clinical problem. The reference book, *Clinical Decision Analysis,* discusses these analyses in full.[2]

REFERENCES

1. Statland BE: *Clinical Decision Levels for Lab Tests*. Oradell, NJ, Medical Economics Books, 1983.

2. Weinstein MC, Fineberg HV: *Clinical Decision Analysis*. Philadelphia, W B Saunders, 1980.

☐ Clinical Problem

ACUTE ABDOMINAL PAIN

Acute or subacute abdominal pain in an adult.

Conditions to be identified

An approach to abdominal pain in adults must focus on differentiating potentially emergent problems that require prompt surgical intervention from those that are best treated without surgery. The following are some of the many conditions that may bring a patient to the office with acute or subacute abdominal pain:

- appendicitis
- acute cholecystitis
- acute or chronic diverticulitis
- acute intermittent porphyria
- acute pancreatitis
- acute urinary tract inflammation
- biliary duct obstruction
- carcinoma of the pancreas
- carcinoma of the stomach
- cholecystitis and cholelithiasis
- chronic relapsing pancreatitis
- ectopic pregnancy
- gastroenteritis
- intermittent intestinal obstruction
- intestinal obstruction
- irritable colon syndrome
- nephrolithiasis
- mesenteric vascular occlusion
- ovarian cyst rupture
- pelvic inflammatory disease (PID)
- peptic ulcer perforation

Degree of urgency

Abdominal pain may portend a serious medical emergency. The major concerns are whether diagnosis or management requires hospitalization and whether the pain is in fact caused by a problem that needs immediate surgical intervention.

Basis of the laboratory diagnosis

Some causes of abdominal pain are associated with characteristic laboratory findings. An increase in the WBC count in association with an elevated sedimentation rate are hallmarks of inflammation. Infection is also associated with a shift of leukocytes to an increased proportion of immature granulocytes (nonsegmented band cells).

Bleeding into the gastrointestinal (GI) tract may produce obvious bloody stools or a positive test for occult blood. Severe bleeding is associated with a decreasing hemoglobin concentration and hematocrit.

Biliary duct obstruction is correlated with increased serum amylase and bilirubin concentrations. Increased amylase levels and a decreased calcium concentration suggest pancreatitis.

Urinary tract infections in adults will generally be associated with an increased number of white cells in the urine and, by definition, a positive urine culture. Pyelonephritis will generally be associated with white cell casts as well as an increased number of white cells in urine.

Gynecologic infections, a common cause of abdominal pain in women during their reproductive years, may be diagnosed with bacterial cultures. Unfortunately a negative culture cannot rule out the diagnosis.

History, physical examination, and previous lab results

A useful operational classification is to divide the problems into those causing acute and those causing chronic or recurrent pain. Acute onset of pain frequently suggests the need for surgical intervention; chronic or recurrent pain is most often relieved by medical therapy. This is obviously a generalization, with the large number of exceptions posing the real challenge in the differential diagnosis.

Inquiry into the onset, duration, nature, localization, and timing of the pain as well as evidence of such associated symptoms as constipation, diarrhea, and flatus are important. Finding a history of chronic abdominal pain with weight loss, anemia, and weakness suggests a malignancy; a history of abdominal pain, fever, and malaise for several weeks might suggest an infectious process such as diverticulitis. Abdominal pain associated with nausea and fever over a number of days is indicative of gastroenteritis; acute abdominal pain without a prodromal period is more suggestive of such diagnoses as simple intestinal obstruction, early appendicitis, biliary colic, or acute pancreatitis.

A history of problems with abdominal pain, such as gallstones or kidney stones, of symptoms associated with PID (painful coitus, vaginal bleeding, or vaginal discharge), and of previous surgical procedures are important in the diagnostic workup.

Physical examination should include documentation of vital signs, including blood pressure, evaluation of postural changes, and temperature. Signs of peritonitis, a change in the character of the bowel sounds, the presence of masses or of free fluid in the abdomen can be important. It is generally prudent to perform rectal and pelvic examinations whenever a surgically treatable cause is being considered.

Initial evaluation

Initial laboratory tests should include a hematocrit or hemoglobin, total and differential white cell count, urinalysis, including the number of red and white cells, detection of glucose and ketone bodies, and a Gram stain of the unspun sediment for bacteria. A stool specimen (from the tip of the examining glove, for example) should be evaluated for occult blood. When considering particular diagnoses, BUN, glucose, amylase, bilirubin, and aminotransferases (ALT and AST) might be indicated.

Follow-up and management tests

Patients with an acute onset of abdominal pain and possible peritoneal signs should be further evaluated in the hospital rather than monitored as outpatients.

When the pain probably does not require immediate surgical intervention, further evaluation might include a more detailed history, physical examination, and additional laboratory tests. In the patient with chronic or recurrent pain, it may be necessary to monitor the course of the signs and symptoms and do appropriate laboratory tests over several subsequent visits.

Pitfalls in test interpretation

In general, lab tests used to evaluate abdominal pain are nonspecific and thus not diagnostic of particular disorders. A number of causes are possible: obtaining the same test result in disorders that require very different management (for example, an elevated white count in acute pancreatitis and in acute appendicitis), or having problems with the test itself (a positive test result for occult blood because of a rectal examination in a menstruating woman). Although many practitioners may think that an increased serum amylase value indicates only pancreatitis, it can also be elevated in other disorders that produce abdominal pain—intestinal obstruction, peptic ulcer, and mesenteric artery thrombosis. The differential diagnosis of an increased amylase value can be very difficult; one helpful nonlaboratory discriminator is the character and radiation of the pain.

Another source of confusion is the variable manifestation of laboratory findings in different patients. For example, older patients who are very ill may not have an increased WBC count even with a potentially life-threatening infection. Younger patients may also have a "normal" total white cell count during the acute phase of a serious infection; but in contrast to older patients, they will generally have a very large number of immature granulocytes. Additional tests, such as the sedimentation rate, may be an important adjunct in clarifying the older patient's differential diagnosis (Chapter 12).

REFERENCE

1. Seward C: *Bedside Diagnosis*. Baltimore, Williams & Wilkins, 1965.

☐ Clinical Problem

ALCOHOLISM

Clinical problem
You suspect that a middle-aged man complaining of memory loss is drinking heavily.

Condition to be identified
Potential alcohol abuse (more than 120 grams of ethanol daily—equivalent to 8 ounces of strong liquor).

Degree of urgency
Problems associated with alcohol abuse are usually chronic, and diagnosis is not of great urgency.[1]

Basis of the laboratory diagnosis
Two tests, the serum gamma-glutamyltransferase (GGT) and the mean red cell corpuscular volume (MCV), have been proposed as useful for detecting excessive alcohol use, but recent studies have shown that neither one is very sensitive. About 30% of individuals who have more than 16 drinks a day or who have been admitted to an alcohol treatment program have abnormal GGT results.[2] Another problem is that a number of medications (including antiepileptic drugs) can cause elevated serum GGT values in the absence of liver disease (Chapter 3).

As for the MCV, the average red cell size difference between nondrinkers and heavy drinkers is small. Although the upper limit of the reference range for MCV varies somewhat from laboratory to laboratory, only about 25% to 30% of heavy drinkers can be expected to have elevated MCV values.[3] Other liver enzyme tests are even less sensitive than the two we've discussed here.

History, physical examination, and previous laboratory tests
Studies have shown that direct inquiry about alcohol use is more effective in detecting abuse than are laboratory tests. Questionnaires and interviewing techniques that take less than a minute have high predictive value and are both sensitive and specific for detecting alcoholism.

Initial evaluation

Of the techniques mentioned in the preceding paragraph, the Brief MAST (Michigan Alcoholism Screening Test), the CAGE (an anagram for key words in the questionnaire), and the Reich interviews have been found most useful. The CAGE interview is based on these key questions[4]:

- Have you ever felt you ought to **C**ut down on your drinking?
- Have people **A**nnoyed you by criticizing your drinking?
- Have you ever felt **G**uilty about your drinking?
- Have you ever had a morning **E**ye-opener?

If you suspect alcohol abuse, it may also be helpful to perform tests used to assess a patient's nutritional status described later in this chapter.

REFERENCES

1. Marks V: Clinical pathology of alcohol. *J Clin Pathol* 1983;36:365-378.

2. Bernadt MW, Mumford J, Taylor C, et al: Comparison of questionnaire and laboratory tests in the detection of excessive drinking and alcoholism. *Lancet* 1982;1:325-328.

3. Eckardt MJ, Ryback RS, Rawlings RR, et al: Biochemical diagnosis of alcoholism. A test of the discriminating capabilities of gamma-glutamyl transpeptidase and mean corpuscular volume. *JAMA* 1981;246:2707-2710.

4. Ewing JA: Detecting alcoholism. The CAGE questionnaire. *JAMA* 1984;252:1905-1907.

☐ Clinical Problem

DIABETES

- Symptoms that suggest diabetes mellitus in an adult.
- Screening for gestational diabetes in a pregnant woman.

Conditions to be identified

- Fasting hyperglycemia in an adult.
- Gestational diabetes.

Degree of urgency

A patient not previously diagnosed as diabetic but with the classic symptoms of polyuria, polydypsia, polyphagia, and weight loss should be evaluated immediately. Patients whose acid-base status cannot be evaluated promptly in the office should be transferred to the hospital for evaluation and treatment. Unfortunately, patients with less classic symptoms can also have significant, potentially dangerous dehydration and acid-base abnormalities, so a blood glucose procedure should be promptly performed in the office to assess the possibility of diabetes mellitus, particularly for older patients.

Because of the potential hazards of a hyperglycemic environment to the fetus, it is essential to screen women for gestational diabetes throughout pregnancy.

Basis of the laboratory diagnosis

In the last decade, the diagnosis of diabetes mellitus in nonpregnant individuals has become more flexible. Finding a fasting blood glucose value greater than 200 mg/dL indicates clinically significant diabetes mellitus. Values between 140 mg/dL and 200 mg/dL can be described as glucose intolerance in some patients (for example, in an 80-year-old patient).

The laboratory diagnosis of gestational diabetes is still based on finding glucose intolerance following a glucose load. Because of changes in how the kidney handles glucose during pregnancy, the standard 100-gram glucose tolerance test (GTT) has a high false-positive rate. Most obstetricians thus use a 50-gram screening GTT with the 100-gram test reserved for women whose one-hour value exceeds 130 mg/dL. Obstetricians today consider a woman to have gestational diabetes if glucose levels exceed 190, 165, and 145 mg/dL at one, two, and three hours, respectively, after a 100-gram load. This approach still gives a measurable false-positive rate, but it is better to treat a few women who do not have the disorder than to miss many who do.

History, physical examination, and previous lab results

By definition, these patients do not have an obvious history of hyperglycemia or diabetes mellitus. Family history of diabetes mellitus (particularly if noninsulin-dependent diabetes is a possibility) can be helpful information, as can a history of large babies or a difficult delivery in pregnant women.

Initial evaluation

In nonpregnant adults being evaluated for diabetes mellitus, a random blood glucose can be further tested if the result is greater than 200 mg/dL—unless the person had a heavy carbohydrate load in the previous two hours. If that's the case and the patient is likely to have diabetes, retest at least two hours later.

In screening for gestational diabetes, the patient should be given a 50-gram glucose load following three days of adequate carbohydrate ingestion and an overnight fast. Blood is collected one hour later, and a result greater than 130 mg/dL is positive.

Follow-up and management tests

A suspicious result from a random glucose assay should be followed up with a fasting GTT the next morning. If the patient is older, appears sick, or has a result greater than 300 mg/dL, however, further evaluation in the office is warranted. In these patients, acidosis (assessing either the serum CO_2 or the serum ketone bodies), hyperkalemia, and dehydration (an elevated BUN or hemoglobin concentration) should be evaluated. We discuss how to help patients reliably manage their own glycemic control in Chapter 16.

As we noted, a positive screen for gestational diabetes should be followed with a second GTT with a 100-gram load (different from the GTT for nonpregnant patients, which now uses a 75-gram load). The patient must have the test in the morning after an overnight fast. Positive results are detailed in the section above on diagnosis.

Pitfalls in test interpretation

The single greatest pitfall in evaluating a blood glucose result is not knowing exactly when the specimen was collected in relation to the last meal. This can be a matter of definition on the patient's part—not considering a bedtime snack a meal, for example. It can also be carelessness by the person collecting the early-morning specimen—assuming that the patient has not had breakfast. It is important to record the time of collection and the time and amount of carbohydrate load when the specimen is collected: This information is essential for accurate interpretation. When collecting a specimen to evaluate symptomatic patients, it is important to find out if they have recently ingested carbohydrates.

If so, they must be rescheduled for specimen collection and be instructed to fast beforehand.

REFERENCES

1. Callaway CW, Rossini AA: Diabetes mellitus, in Branch WT, *Office Practice of Medicine*. Philadelphia, WB Saunders, 1982.

2. National Diabetes Data Group: Classification and diagnosis of diabetes mellitus and other categories of glucose intolerance. *Diabetes* 1979;28:1039-1057.

☐ Clinical Problem

GONORRHEA

- A patient with a discharge that may be caused by gonorrhea.
- Evaluation of possible gonorrhea in an asymptomatic contact.

Conditions to be identified

- Gonorrhea.
- Nongonococcal urethritis.

Degree of urgency

Because of the rapidity with which gonorrhea can spread through a community, particularly a closed community, the condition should be diagnosed as quickly as possible. All contacts of anyone found to have gonorrhea should also be evaluated promptly.

Basis of the laboratory diagnosis

Ideally, finding *Neisseria gonorrhoeae* in culture with subsequent confirmation is the definitive diagnostic test. Unfortunately, the test is time-consuming (usually two or three days until isolation with an additional day for confirmation), and a single culture does not always show the organism, even when it is known to be present. Consequently, other approaches to diagnosis and confirmation have been used. In men, the most common symptom is urethral discharge, so the most expedient approach is to prepare a Gram-stained slide of discharge and look for gram-negative, intracellular diplococci in polymorphic granulocytes.

This approach is not effective in women because normal vaginal and cervical flora includes a variety of nongonococcal gram-negative diplococci. Nor are immunologic tests feasible since antibodies tend to persist long after the acute infection, and a positive test merely indicates contact with the organism sometime in the indeterminate past.

Approaches to shortening the time needed to confirm the diagnosis have focused on methods that do not require incubating the isolates. The classic methods use sugars in the growth medium to differentiate the organism from those that are morphologically identical but different in terms of clinical importance. These methods also use immunofluorescence techniques, which are impractical for most office laboratories because of the equipment cost and technical skill required to perform the tests.

Finally, the emerging gonococcal resistance to penicillin is becoming an important problem. It can be recognized simultaneously with the confirmatory tests by incubating the organism in a culture medium with penicillin and an indicator that changes color when the penicillin is inactivated by penicillinase.

History, physical examination, and previous lab results

Contact with someone infected with gonorrhea, urethral discharge in a man, or purulent cervical discharge in a woman are all reasons to pursue the diagnosis. A history of multiple sex partners and previous infections with gonorrhea or other venereal infections should also suggest the possibility of gonococcal infection. In a venereal disease clinic or related general practices, it may even be appropriate to consider the possibility of gonorrhea in all patients because of the high rate of asymptomatic infection among women (and, perhaps, among men as well) and consider screening cultures for all patients.

Initial evaluation

Diagnosis begins with a urethral smear in men and a cervical culture in women. Preparing and interpreting a Gram-stained urethral smear takes some skill, and the inexperienced practitioner should not undertake them because of the high potential for false-positive and false-negative results. For the unskilled practitioner, we recommend training in a local laboratory or venereal disease clinic or using other diagnostic approaches (such as culture). In areas with a relatively high incidence of penicillin-resistant *N. gonorrhoeae,* the initial evaluation should include testing all isolates for resistance.

Follow-up and management tests

As we noted, clinical follow-up includes evaluating symptomatic and asymptomatic contacts of the infected person. If an infection does not respond to initial treatment, additional cultures should be done and tested for penicillin resistance (since these organisms tend to be multiply resistant to antibiotics other than penicillin). If the laboratory saves primary culture plates for several days after reporting the results, it would save time to test these organisms for resistance to penicillin.

Despite the availability of several new tests on the market, the office diagnosis of *Chlamydia* remains a process of exclusion. If the gonococcal culture and the clinical picture suggest nongonococcal urethritis, a therapeutic trial with tetracycline or erythromycin is indicated.

Pitfalls in test interpretation

The diagnostic sensitivity of a test for gonorrhea depends, first and foremost, on the specimen collection technique. The organism is not uniformly distributed over the cervix and the cervical os or in the urethra. It is focally distributed, and vigorous swabbing of the culture site is essential to capture gonococci in medium to low concentrations.

In addition, a single culture is less than fully effective in capturing the organism, so authorities recommend that a second one be obtained from the same site (the cervix and urethra are preferred for the initial culture) or from another (rectum, urethra, or vagina). It is possible to plate the second specimen onto the same culture plate as the first without significant loss of the sensitivity of using two plates. It must be remembered that sites other than the cervix or urethra—the oral pharynx and tonsils, for example—should also be cultured in homosexuals.

Inasmuch as the organisms tend to be absorbed into the center of a cotton swab, they are less available for deposit on the culture plate. Calgonite swabs are preferred; their tips tend to disintegrate when moist, releasing the absorbed organisms and making them available for deposit on the medium. The organism is also very fragile; it does not tolerate ambient room temperature or humidity very well, and it requires prompt plating and incubation in CO_2 at or near 37 C. Even when these conditions are met, *N. gonorrhoeae* will not be identified in all infected patients. The yield is estimated to vary from 80% to 98% when using two specimens for culture.[1]

The culture systems being promoted for use in the office laboratory have some additional pitfalls. First, the office laboratory may perform fewer tests and thus keep the medium longer; it is therefore necessary to ensure that the medium is viable. Dehydration would reduce its ability to support growth.

Some systems have moisture added to the culture packet to initiate a reaction producing CO_2. Again, dehydrated media will prevent this reaction; there will be a markedly reduced yield and thus a high false-negative rate. It is essential to inspect the media before use and discard any plates that seem to have growth or media pulled away from the edges or bottom.

The last important point is spreading the organisms over the medium. Using conventional plates, the initial sample should be rolled across two quadrants of the plate. Then a flamed loop should be used to spread the organism into the third quadrant, and after reflaming the loop, to spread the organism from the third quadrant into the fourth. Most portable media used to isolate *N. gonorrhoeae* have a much smaller surface for spreading the organisms—which is critical to the primary identification. The swab should therefore be rolled across the short side at one end of the unit, forming a very narrow band. Then a flamed loop can be used to spread the organisms a number of times from this narrow band at one end parallel to the longer dimension of the culture unit. These techniques maximize the yield of these otherwise fragile organisms.

REFERENCES

1. Judson FN, Werness BA: Combining cervical and anal-canal specimens for gonorrhea on a single culture plate. *J Clin Microbiol* 1980;12:216-219.

General references

Washington JA: Medical bacteriology, in Henry JB (ed), *Clinical Diagnosis and Management by Laboratory Methods,* ed 17. Philadelphia, WB Saunders, 1984.

Woo B, Bruce M, Branch WT: Penile discharge and urethritis, in Branch WT (ed), *Office Practice of Medicine.* Philadelphia, WB Saunders, 1982.

☐ Clinical Problem

HYPERTENSION

A patient is newly discovered to have diastolic hypertension.

Basis of the laboratory diagnosis

Laboratory evaluation of hypertension has three major objectives: 1) to screen for its secondary, possibly reversible forms; 2) to ascertain the degree of end-organ damage it may have caused; and 3) to identify patients at high risk for developing cardiovascular complications.

Secondary hypertension occurs in about 5% of all patients seen in the clinical setting. Among its prominent causes that can be identified by history, physical examination, or laboratory tests are Cushing's syndrome, coarctation of the aorta, pheochromocytoma, drugs, primary aldosteronism, renal disease, and renovascular disease. Renal insufficiency and cardiac hypertrophy may also result from prolonged or severe hypertension. The risk of atherosclerotic disease in patients with hypertension is greater when there is also a history of smoking, hypercholesterolemia, diabetes, or obesity.

Degree of urgency

In a newly identified hypertensive patient, a diastolic pressure of 135 mm Hg or higher, retinal hemorrhages, or papilledema strongly suggests that hospitalization is necessary for prompt evaluation and treatment. Caution in such patients is indicated since drastic drops in blood pressure could cause stroke in someone with a history of transient cerebral ischemic attacks.

History and physical examination

Both can clarify the etiology of the hypertension, likely end-organ damage from prolonged high blood pressure, and the risk of atherosclerotic disease. Patients at a somewhat higher risk for secondary hypertension include the younger age group (under 35 years) and those with a rapid onset of elevated blood pressure, severe hypertension, poor response to past therapy, and no family history of hypertension. Specific clues include the following:

Cushing's syndrome. Classic facial appearance with virilism and hirsutism occasionally noted.

Coarctation of the aorta. A different blood pressure in the arm compared with the leg, which is first suggested by simultaneously palpating the radial-femoral pulse.

Drug-induced hypertension. A history of using amphetamines, oral contraceptives, estrogens, corticosteroids, licorice, or thyroid medication.

Hyperthyroidism. Systolic pressure greater than 160 mm Hg, but diastolic pressure less than 90 mm Hg. This systolic hypertension might also be associated with aortic valvular insufficiency or arteriovenous fistula.

Pheochromocytoma. A history of headaches, palpitations, tachycardia, and unprovoked sweating.

Primary hyperaldosteronism. Hypertension in association with hypokalemia without a history of diuretic therapy or gastrointestinal (GI) fluid losses.

Renovascular disease. This should be suspected in a young woman or an elderly patient with arteriosclerosis, especially with sudden onset, an abdominal bruit, and no family history of hypertension.

Initial evaluation

The following tests are probably indicated in all patients first seen for hypertension: chest x-ray studies, ECG, blood urea nitrogen (BUN), creatinine, cholesterol, fasting glucose, potassium, routine urinalysis, sodium, and fasting triglyceride.

Primary renal disease will often be supported by an abnormal urinalysis. Proteinuria, casts, or high urinary RBC or WBC values may be present. How closely the renal insufficiency is related to or a cause of the hypertension is indicated by elevated BUN and creatinine values. Decreased serum potassium values (less than 3.6 mmol/L) or elevated serum sodium values would suggest further evaluation for primary hyperaldosteronism.

Cardiovascular risk would be indicated by elevated fasting blood glucose, increased serum cholesterol values, and ECG changes. The latter may also suggest cardiac damage related to the hypertension.

Elevated BUN values (greater than 40 mg/dL) or increased serum creatinine values (greater than 4 mg/dL) would suggest hospitalization to evaluate the patient for possible renal disease. In such patients it is prudent to avoid lowering the diastolic pressure below 105 mm Hg; this risks reduced renal flow promoting further BUN or creatinine elevations.

Identifying patients whose hypertension is potentially reversible is extremely important. This applies to only a fraction of the hypertensives you will see, but if even a few can avoid a lifetime of medication with its attendant problems, it will justify this effort. The clues from the history and physical examination assume even greater importance in such cases.

- Evaluating for Cushing's disease would include an 8 AM serum cortisol test, with a value above 25 μg/dL strongly suggesting the disease. Following up with a urinary free cortisol test, values greater than 100 μg of free cortisol per 24-hour collection would support the Cushing's diagnosis, which is usually confirmed with the dexamethasone suppression test. The patient is given 1 mg of dexamethasone at 11 PM; a morning serum cortisol value above 10 μg/dL is confirmatory. A high-dose (8 mg) dexamethasone suppression test can then be done to distinguish between adrenal hyperplasia and adrenal tumor.

- The laboratory diagnosis of pheochromocytoma begins with determining urinary levels of metanephrines. Values below 1.3 mg per 24-hour collection along with normal vanillylmandelic acid (VMA) values exclude the diagnosis in 95% of the cases. Values above 2.5 mg per 24 hours confirm a catecholamine-producing tumor provided there is no possibility of analytical interference from drugs or diet. Normal metanephrine values when there is a high suspicion of multiple endocrine adenomatosis Type II would suggest ordering the more specific urinary catecholamine or plasma catecholamine test along with localizing tests. Angiography can usually locate the tumors, which can then be surgically excised.

- A decreased serum potassium value suggests primary hyperaldosteronism. The hypokalemia should not be ascribed to diuretic therapy or GI losses. Clinical clues supporting hyperaldosteronism include muscle weakness and nocturnal polyuria. A urinary potassium level greater than 30 mmol per 24 hours indicates mineralocorticoid-induced hypertension. The presumptive diagnosis here is based on elevated plasma aldosterone values and suppressed plasma renin activity (PRA).

To make PRA determinations more accurate, we recommend mild renin stimulation before measurement. This is done by giving 40 to 80 mg of furosemide orally followed by four hours of standing. An alternative approach is 40 mg furosemide intravenously followed by a half hour of standing. A stimulated PRA value of less than 1 ng/mL/hr suggests excessive salt intake, low renin essential hypertension, or perhaps mineralocorticoid secondary hypertension. Elevated plasma aldosterone values would substantiate primary mineralocorticoid-induced hypertension. Alternatively, a stimulated PRA value greater than 5 ng/mL/hr indicates renin-dependent hypertension, and the patient should be evaluated for renovascular disease.

Follow-up and management tests

Monitoring the patient treated for hypertension involves assessing the efficacy of therapy as well as noting the degree of end-organ damage. Thus routine blood pressure readings are generally indicated. Repeated urinalysis and monitoring BUN, creatinine, and serum potassium values are necessary to detect early signals of renal insufficiency.

Pitfalls in test interpretation

VMA: The reference (normal) interval for VMA is less than 6.8 mg per 24 hours, but increased values may be related to drug intake or diet. Ingesting vanilla, bananas, coffee, tea, or chocolate causes elevated values. Chemical interferences have been noted with anileridine, caffeine, methenamine mandelate, methocarbamol, and salicylates. In addition, exercise stress may also cause an increase in VMA values. In these situations, the more specific catecholamine test would be helpful.

PRA: PRA values have many preanalytical sources of variation. Many commonly used antihypertensive medications, for example, affect PRA. These medications may thus have to be withdrawn for at least two weeks before testing for secondary hypertension. It is also meaningless to measure PRA within six months of using oral contraceptives because of pill-induced vagaries in these levels. A high-sodium diet may often obscure differences in PRA values. Renin specimens generally require special handling techniques: Blood must be drawn into chilled tubes containing EDTA, and the plasma must be separated in a cold centrifuge before assay. Falsely low PRA values may occur if these instructions are not carefully followed.

REFERENCES
1. Howanitz JH, Howanitz PJ: Evaluation of endocrine function, in Henry JB (ed) *Clinical Diagnosis and Management by Laboratory Methods*. Philadelphia, WB Saunders, 1983.
2. Solomen HS: Hypertension, in Branch WT (ed) *Office Practice of Medicine*. Philadelphia, WB Saunders, 1982.

☐ Clinical Problem

NUTRITIONAL ASSESSMENT

A college student who has been eating a strict vegetarian diet complains of feeling tired.

Conditions to be identified

- Malnutrition.
- Nutritional anemia.

Degree of urgency

This problem is probably chronic, and diagnosis is not urgent.

Basis of the laboratory diagnosis

Laboratory testing is most useful in identifying protein-deficiency malnutrition, which usually accompanies calorie deprivation but can also occur with adequate caloric intake. Calorie malnutrition can cause a protein loss as gluconeogenesis consumes endogenous protein. This can in turn lead to a need for more dietary protein, which, if not met, can cause protein malnutrition.

Vitamin and mineral deficiencies are more difficult to assess in the office laboratory. There are only a few well-established tests for detecting them, notably those for iodine (indirectly), iron, folate, and vitamin B_{12}.

A protein deficiency decreases muscle mass, the synthesis of such serum proteins as albumin and transferrin, and lymphocyte production. Measuring these indices can give some indication of protein nutritional status.

History, physical examination, and previous laboratory tests

A radical change in diet, a recent weight loss greater than 10% of the patient's usual weight, or a weight lower than 80% of ideal body weight suggests a nutritional basis for the problem. Such physical findings as pallor, thin skin, and dry brittle hair also suggest malnutrition, but many individuals do not show these signs even in clinically significant malnutrition. Arm circumference and triceps skin folds are helpful measurements, but they must be done by an experienced person. Weight loss from severe malnutrition may, for a time, be obscured by edema associated with electrolyte abnormalities, renal failure, or cardiac disease.

Initial evaluation

A number of laboratory tests can give indirect evidence of malnutrition. No single test can diagnose the condition, however, so a group of tests must be performed and evaluated together. One such group for evaluating calorie malnutrition includes the 24-hour urine creatinine, serum albumin and transferrin concentrations, and total blood lymphocyte count.

The 24-hour urine creatinine excretion test, used to indicate lean body (muscle) mass, requires the patient to refrain from eating meat for a period of time before and during collection. In addition, the collection must be complete and the volume measurement accurate. For this reason, some authors recommend averaging the creatinine excretion results of a 72-hour collection. Using published tables, the creatinine excretion rate and the body height can be used to estimate the lean body mass. The amount of creatinine excreted by a healthy adult is 1,200 mg to 1,600 mg per 24 hours, with males averaging 200 mg more than females. A result below 800 mg per 24 hours would suggest a severely decreased lean body mass.

Serum albumin can be a useful indicator of nutritional status. A concentration of less than 3.4 g/dL suggests poor nutrition when no other causes of depressed albumin production, such as liver disease or nephrotic syndrome, exist. Transferrin, which is decreased in malnutrition, can also be useful in diagnosing malnutrition. Unfortunately, its concentration is also increased during acute inflammation, in several stress-related conditions, and in iron-deficiency anemia. The serum ferritin concentration is depressed in association with the anemia of chronic disease and should not be used to assess nutritional status under these conditions. Reduced BUN, cholesterol, and triglyceride concentrations are consistent with but not diagnostic of malnutrition.

A depressed total lymphocyte count (fewer than 1,500 cells/μL) suggests poor nutrition. The lymphocyte count is affected by such clinical conditions as viral and bacterial infections, malignancy, collagen vascular disease, or steroid therapy, however, so they should be excluded before this measurement can truly indicate nutritional status. Other hematologic studies, such as hemoglobin, hematocrit, and red cell indices are not particularly useful as primary indicators of nutritional status, but may suggest nutritional deficiencies that result in anemia.

In summary, the laboratory approach to diagnosing calorie malnutrition requires a multiple test approach because individual tests lack specificity and sensitivity.

Follow-up and management tests

The tests we've discussed will gradually return to normal values as nutritional status improves. Serum albumin, with its long half-life, is not useful for following rapid changes associated with nutritional therapy. Transferrin has a shorter half-life and can be a more sensitive test for changing nutritional status. But certain nonlaboratory indicators such as weight gain and a change in the patient's sense of well-being are probably much more useful in assessing clinical improvement.

Pitfalls in test interpretation

The tests used in nutritional assessment are only indirect indicators, and their results cannot make a diagnosis by themselves. Furthermore, they are not specific, and they can be influenced by a variety of factors, including concurrent disease, stress, and malfunction of such organs as the kidneys, heart, and liver. Laboratory evaluation of nutritional status thus requires a multiple testing approach, one of which we have described.

Although outside the scope of this discussion, nutritional deficiency and weight loss may be early signs of such serious disease as renal problems, malabsorption, and other disorders (in-

cluding occult malignancies) with these systemic manifestations.
It's important to consider these conditions if other causes do not
become obvious.

REFERENCES

1. Campbell JA: Nutritional evaluation of hospital patients. *Lab Med*
1984;15:666-669.

2. Labbe R (ed): Symposium of laboratory assessment of nutritional
status. *Clin Lab Med* 1981;1:(4).

☐ Clinical Problem

PREADMISSION TESTING

Laboratory testing is required before elective surgery.

Conditions to be identified

- Potential bleeding problem.
- Presence of infection.
- The status of major organ systems.

Degree of urgency

Results should be available before admission, consistent with hospital regulations.

History, physical examination, and previous lab results

In patients undergoing surgery, it is imperative to know whether
the patient has any bleeding tendencies or an unsuspected infection. The patient should be specifically questioned about any
bleeding problems following circumcision, tonsillectomy, dental
extractions, or a major operation or trauma. The questioner
should also ask about spontaneous hemorrhages into the skin or
mucus membranes (including nosebleeds) and into the joints.
Medical history is a far more sensitive indicator of bleeding tendencies than laboratory tests are.

Many medications are metabolized by the kidney or liver,
and it is thus important to know the functional status of these
organs. Morbidity from other clinical problems is important information for the anesthetist and the surgeon. Signs and symp-

toms of current or recent infections should also be carefully sought (a history of dysuria, fever, chills, or diarrhea, for example). A baseline profile of certain laboratory tests can be significant in establishing the patient's own reference range (Chapter 4) to facilitate the evaluation of test results during the postoperative period.

Initial evaluation

Preadmission laboratory tests must be individually customized depending on the patient's age and the problem to be diagnosed or treated during the hospital stay. Tests helpful in a preoperative evaluation include a total WBC count, hematocrit or hemoglobin, and a urinalysis screen with a reagent strip that includes a test for leukocyte esterase. In patients scheduled for major surgery, BUN, bilirubin, prothrombin time (PT) and perhaps the partial thromboplastin time (PTT), serum alkaline phosphatase (ALP), and aspartate aminotransferase (AST, SGOT) should also be determined.

Other preoperative testing will be dictated by the patient's unique problems. The routine use of large profiles of laboratory testing before or at admission should be discouraged. The purpose of preoperative laboratory testing is to uncover conditions that might change the patient's management or cancel the surgery, to find other morbid conditions that must be evaluated, or to assess an organ system's status that would be critical in the patient's care. Preadmission testing should not be used to screen for asymptomatic or presymptomatic disease unrelated to the problems at hand.

Follow-up and management tests

If an abnormal WBC count (above 12,000 or below 4,000 cells per microliter) is found, a differential count should be performed. An elevated white cell count with a large proportion of immature granulocytes might suggest an infection or at least the possibility of a significant focus of inflammation. Determining the sedimentation rate might be useful in selected patients with the possibility of infection or inflammation but poorly reactive defenses.

Finding pyuria, with either leukocyte esterase reagent strips or microscopic analysis of urinary sediment, suggests the possibility of an asymptomatic urinary tract infection, which should be confirmed with a urine culture. This assumes a clean-voided urine specimen, of course (Chapter 3). An increase in serum BUN suggests the possibility of renal insufficiency, which may be clarified with a serum creatinine determination, but might actually require a creatinine clearance test.

Abnormalities in the PT or PTT suggest the possibility of bleeding problems, and they demand further evaluation before surgery. This could be resolved by finding out specifically that the patient has had major surgery in the past without incident. Otherwise, further testing might be required, including tests to differentiate procoagulant deficiencies from circulating anticoagulants. Abnormalities in the screening tests for liver dysfunction (AST, ALP, or bilirubin) should be noted, and the patient questioned further to define the nature of the problem, particularly if it was unsuspected. It is especially important to identify individuals with hepatitis so that suitable precautions can be exercised to protect hospital employees and other patients from exposure to the infection.

Pitfalls in test interpretation

Using laboratory tests in this group of patients will produce a predictable number of false-positive results because of analytic variation or the laboratory definition of reference ranges (Chapter 4). Since we define normality as only 95% of a healthy population, the other 5% will have an abnormal result for each test in the profile. Thus, as we noted, preadmission testing should not be used to screen for disease. Nevertheless, the significance of an abnormal result in clinically relevant testing should be evaluated.

Because of the technical competence required for a microscopic urinalysis, it is subject to a high degree of analytic variation. In the office setting, the urine reagent strip can be confidently substituted as a prescreen to indicate which sediments should be further evaluated.

□ Clinical Problem

PREGNANCY TESTING

A woman of child-bearing age complains of amenorrhea or lower abdominal pain.

Conditions to be identified
- Normal pregnancy.
- Amenorrhea due to a condition other than pregnancy, such as malnutrition, an unusual exercise program, or endocrine abnormalities.
- Ectopic pregnancy.
- Exclusion of ectopic pregnancy as a cause of abdominal pain or dysfunctional uterine bleeding.

Degree of urgency

Ectopic pregnancy is a potential emergency. Until recently, 6% to 11% of maternal deaths in the United States have been caused by ruptured ectopic pregnancies. The current mortality rate is 1.4 deaths per 1,000 diagnosed ectopic pregnancies.[1]

Basis of the laboratory diagnosis

Diagnosing a normal pregnancy involves the detection of human chorionic gonadotropin (hCG), a pregnancy hormone produced by the chorionic villae of the placenta. The hormone functions to prolong the life of the corpus luteum until the placenta produces enough estrogens and progestogens to satisfy the needs of pregnancy. Today's pregnancy tests use immunologic methods to detect intact hCG or its beta subunit (Chapter 15).

History, physical examination, and previous lab results

In most cases, the physician is responding to the question of pregnancy from amenorrheic, otherwise healthy women. It is important to ask about previous ectopic pregnancy, abortion, the use of an intrauterine device (IUD), pelvic inflammatory disease, chronic or acute salpingitis, and any surgical procedures on the fallopian tubes, all of which increase the ectopic pregnancy risk.

The physician is often faced with a young woman with a history of abdominal pain or dysfunctional uterine bleeding in whom the issue of an extrauterine pregnancy must be excluded.

Although a recent menstrual history and inquiry into the predisposing factors just mentioned can be helpful, no single one is conclusive, and the diagnosis of pregnancy rests on determining the hCG concentration in blood or urine.

Initial evaluation

A normal pregnancy can be diagnosed with almost any currently available urine or blood test. Except for certain considerations that we'll discuss in a moment, cost and convenience should be of paramount importance.

By contrast, diagnosing an ectopic pregnancy requires the most sensitive test, either urine or blood, in order to detect the lower expected concentration of hCG (compared with levels of the same gestational age in a normal pregnancy). A negative result with any test, however, does not rule out either a normal or an ectopic pregnancy.

Follow-up and management tests

Follow-up testing in amenorrhea can be repeated in seven to 10 days. Because of the rapid increase of hCG during early pregnancy, the second test will generally be positive if the patient is pregnant, but further testing may still be required. We'll discuss interfering factors shortly.

In someone with a positive hCG result, confirming the diagnosis of an ectopic pregnancy requires further evaluation with abdominal ultrasound and possibly diagnostic culdocentesis, laparoscopy, or laparotomy. When these findings are equivocal, further follow-up with serum β hCG tests every other day to look for the expected doubling of hCG concentration can be helpful, along with clinical evaluation.

In someone with a negative result and suspected pregnancy, continued surveillance and testing are necessary to confirm the diagnosis. Should the attending physician believe that the risk of ectopic pregnancy is very high in an acutely ill patient, an abdominal ultrasound and exploratory laparoscopy or laparotomy may be required to make the diagnosis.

Pitfalls in test interpretation

Normal pregnancy. Some of today's pregnancy tests set the threshold value for a positive test at a level of hCG expected at or before a menstrual period (Figure 5-3). But many spontaneous

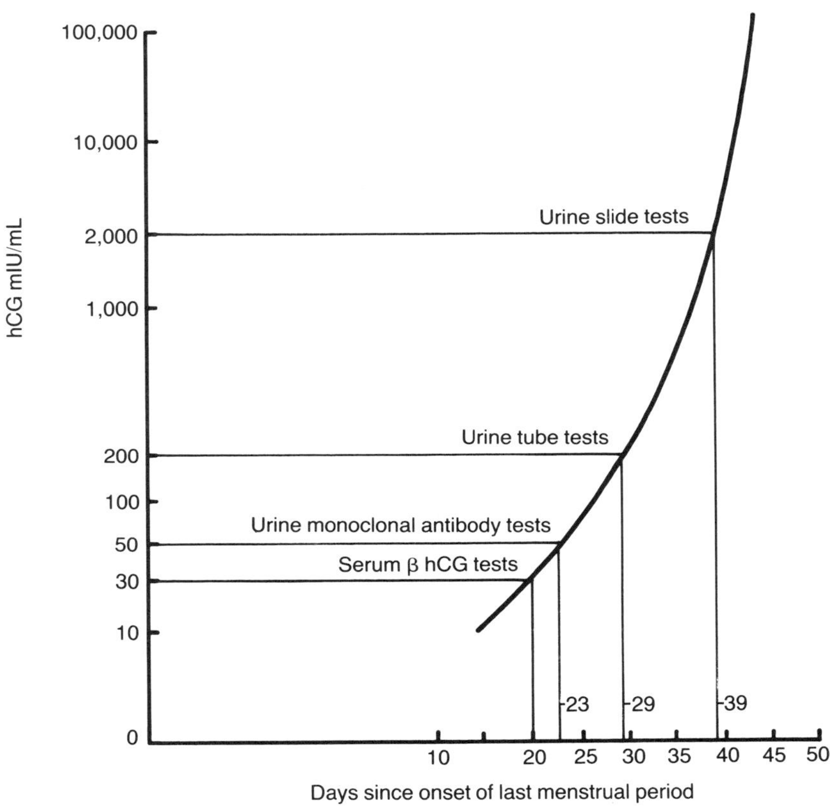

abortions occur in the first month of pregnancy. It is thus important to use a test with a threshold value of hCG expected at least seven days after the missed period to reduce such false-positive diagnoses. A urine test with a threshold value of 200 to 300 mIU/mL is a reasonable approach to this problem with a repeat test in seven to 14 days if the first result is negative. The serum β hCG is too sensitive (and usually more expensive) and should not be used to diagnose normal pregnancy until at least seven to 10 days after the missed period.

Ectopic pregnancy remains a diagnostic challenge in spite of markedly improved testing tools. As noted, the diagnosis is complicated by the fact that the hCG secretion is reduced because of the smaller placenta caused by its limited blood supply and retarded growth in the abnormal implantation site. A small fraction of patients later proven to have an ectopic pregnancy will, in fact, have negative serum and urine hCG tests when they are first tested. The clinician should use the most sensitive test available that also gives timely results.

Some of today's highly specific urine tests (double monoclonal antibody tests with a colorimetric reaction and little or no LH cross-reactivity) can be used below the threshold limit for a normal pregnancy. With these tests, any color development probably indicates hCG.

Serum β hCG. There is generally little or no cross-reactivity between β-specific hCG antibodies and other glycoprotein hormones, but the clinician should be aware of the operating characteristics of the test used in the office, hospital, and referral laboratories.

Urine hCG. These methods are subject to a number of factors that can affect result interpretation. For example, a negative result with a dilute random specimen should be repeated because the test is sensitive to the concentration of urinary hCG. Many laboratories test for a low urine specific gravity (a cause of false-negative results) and in latex or red cell agglutination methods, for a high urine protein concentration (a cause of false-positive results). Slide tests, which are slightly less sensitive, are not recommended because the critically important tilting required for mixing them leads to higher false-positive and false-negative rates.

Home pregnancy tests. Women using these kits have been shown to produce 4% to 5% false-positive results,[2] a markedly higher rate than that of trained professionals. Although the package insert usually advises the patient that the test is not definitive and she should consult her physician, many women rely on the results and suffer unnecessarily. Consequently, if patients want to use these tests at home, they should be tutored in the proper technique for analysis and interpretation (Chapter 17).

REFERENCES

1. MacKay HT, Hughes JM, Hogue CR: Ectopic pregnancy in the United States, 1979-1980. *CDC Surveillance Summaries* 1984;33:1SS-7SS.

2. e.p.t. plus Early Pregnancy Test, *Physicians' Desk Reference for Nonprescription Drugs*, 6th ed., Oradell, NJ, Medical Economics, 1985, p 742.

General references

Kreig AF, Wenk RE: Pregnancy tests and evaluation of placental function, in Henry JB (ed), *Clinical Diagnosis and Management by Laboratory Methods,* 17th ed, Philadelphia, WB Saunders, 1984.

Speroff L, Glass RH, Kase NG: *Clinical Gynecologic Endocrinology & Infertility,* 3rd ed, Baltimore, Williams & Wilkins, 1983.

☐ Clinical Problem

SORE THROAT

A child has acute pharyngitis.

Conditions to be identified

- Pharyngitis due to group A beta-hemolytic streptococcus.
- Viral pharyngitis.
- Infectious mononucleosis.

Basis of the laboratory diagnosis

Serious sequelae of infections with group A beta-hemolytic streptococci include glomerular nephritis, rheumatic fever, and peritonsillar abscess. Antibiotic therapy can prevent the last two, but not the first. On the other hand, a small proportion of patients will have allergic reactions associated with penicillin therapy. It would be unfortunate to produce an allergic reaction in someone whose pharyngitis was caused by an organism—such as a virus—that is not susceptible to antibiotics.

Streptococci can also be recovered in the pharynx of perhaps 20% to 30% of asymptomatic individuals at times of endemic disease. During epidemics, the asymptomatic carrier rate is even higher. Given this information and the fact that accurately culturing and identifying group A beta-hemolytic streptococci require considerable skill and experience, some investigators have recommended other approaches to diagnosis or treatment.[1-3]

One strategy suggests that when there is epidemic or moderately high incidence of endemic infections, all symptomatic patients should be treated with penicillin. When the rate of positive throat cultures is between 5% and 20% of the patient population, treatment should be based on culture results. When there is an extremely low rate of positive throat cultures—less than 5%—penicillin therapy is not recommended. More recently, immuno-diagnostic methods have been developed for the rapid identification of group A beta-hemolytic streptococci.[4]

History, physical examination, and previous laboratory tests

Using such a testing and therapy strategy depends on knowing the incidence of group A beta-hemolytic streptococcus pharyngitis in the community. Patient contact with proven cases of streptococcal pharyngitis or a history of rheumatic fever will influence the decision to start therapy. Suggestive physical findings include high fever, tonsillar exudate, tender, swollen neck lymph nodes, or scarlatiniform rash. Laboratory findings of leukocytosis and a shift to the left support a bacterial source, while leukopenia, relative lymphocytosis, and atypical lymphocytes suggest nonbacterial causes.

Initial evaluation

The most cost-effective strategy will usually be to presume there is streptococcal infection and treat the patient without confirmatory tests. If laboratory tests are done, a throat culture carefully obtained from the tonsillar pillars and posterior pharyngeal wall is essential (Chapter 14 gives specific information about testing systems). A CBC at the initial visit is usually unnecessary.

Follow-up and management tests

If the pharyngitis does not respond to therapy and the patient remains symptomatic, a viral cause should be considered. It may be advisable to perform tests for infectious mononucleosis (Chapter 15).

Pitfalls in test interpretation

The high asymptomatic carrier rate for group A beta-hemolytic streptococcus markedly diminishes the value of throat cultures in diagnosing streptococcal pharyngitis. False-negative results can occur if the specimen is not properly collected. As mentioned, specimens must be taken from the tonsillar pillars and posterior pharynx, which is uncomfortable for the patient and particularly difficult in a small child. Negative cultures yielding minimal growth indicate unsatisfactory specimen collection or a problem in the laboratory. The bacitracin A disk for differentiating group A beta-hemolytic streptococcus from other organisms lacks specificity, and its error rate is estimated at 5% to 15%. Although the rapid immunodiagnostic tests for group A beta-hemolytic streptococci are widely used, no studies have demonstrated their effectiveness and reliability in diagnosing significant infection.

REFERENCES

1. Tompkins RK, Burnes DC, Cable WE: An analysis of the cost effectiveness of pharyngitis management and acute rheumatic fever prevention. *Ann Intern Med* 1977;86:481-492.

2. Bisno AL: Therapeutic strategies for the prevention of rheumatic fever (editorial). *Ann Intern Med* 1977;86:494-496.

3. Pantell RH: Cost-effectiveness of pharyngitis management and prevention of rheumatic fever (editorial). *Ann Intern Med* 1977;86:497-499.

4. Rapid office tests for streptococcal pharyngitis. *The Medical Letter* 1985;27:49-51.

☐ Clinical Problem

STOOL OCCULT BLOOD

A patient has a positive test for occult blood in the stool.

Conditions to be identified

Colorectal cancer.

Degree of urgency

Although a colorectal malignancy has probably been present for years before its discovery, the practitioner must evaluate the problem as expeditiously as possible. This is largely because of the patient's fear of cancer after finding out about the positive test result.

Basis of the laboratory diagnosis

Colorectal carcinoma is one of the most common malignancies in adult men and women. The frequency of diagnosis in adults older than 50 is about 1 per 1,000 individuals annually. The prognosis and survival rate depend directly on the stage of disease when diagnosed. The five-year survival rate varies from 90% when the lymph nodes are negative and the lesion is limited to the mucosa, to 15% with positive nodes and extension throughout the entire bowel wall, including the serosa.[1] Early detection is thus of unquestionable value.

When malignancy is detected before the onset of symptoms, 80% of the patients will not have nodal involvement, and their five-year survival rate will range from 70% to 90%. We recommend annual stool occult blood testing for all asymptomatic, over-50 adults.

Individually packaged test kits for occult blood, which are now available from several manufacturers, are widely used in the office setting. This procedure is based on the guaiac-peroxide reaction and should be positive in the presence of blood. According to a series of studies of patients with diagnosed, biopsy-proven, colorectal carcinoma, a single test for occult blood was positive in about 40% of all patients and in 33% of those with cancer limited to the mucosa (Duke's Stage A).[1]

In the past year or two, stool occult blood tests packaged and designed for home use have become available. The results of such testing should be discussed between doctor and patient, especially in terms of the reliability of such assays and the implications of a positive result.

History and physical examination

A history of black tarry stools or of overt blood in the feces would demand further investigation to rule out malignancy. A change in bowel habits (constipation, diarrhea, size or texture of stool) also suggests a possible colorectal malignancy. Increased risk has been related to diet, a family history of colonic carcinoma, familial polyposis, and ulcerative colitis starting before age 25.

Initial evaluation

Because of a fairly high rate of false-positive screening tests, it is essential to confirm a positive finding before doing more invasive diagnostic procedures. Patient preparation and sample collection are critical factors in maximizing the reliability of stool occult blood tests. Current recommendations are to collect two specimens from different parts of the stool each day for three days. The ideal diet, starting 24 hours before the first stool collection and lasting throughout the period, is high residue and meat-free. Vitamin C and aspirin should not be consumed. Each specimen should be tested within two to four days of its collection.

Follow-up and management tests

Confirmation of occult blood in the stool should prompt the clinician to investigate further. This includes proctosigmoidoscopy, which detects up to 50% of all colorectal carcinomas, followed by a properly performed barium enema, including air contrast studies, which should identify up to 90% of malignant colorectal lesions. Air-contrast studies are more sensitive than full-column studies for small lesions, but there is a greater risk of missing larger lesions.

Patients with colon cancer and elevated carcinoembryonic antigen (CEA) should be monitored for recurrence using the serum CEA test. This test should be done every two months for the first year and then every six months. A CEA value above 5 ng/mL in a patient known to have carcinoma of the colon suggests recurrence. CEA testing should never be used as a screening tool, however. It is, at best, a monitoring tool of minor value in confirming the diagnosis of colon cancer in the symptomatic patient.

Pitfalls in test interpretation

Both clinical and analytic problems can produce false-positive results for occult blood screening and confirmatory tests. In fact, a number of studies have shown that only 5% to 10% of individuals with positive test results actually have carcinoma of the colon (a 90% to 95% false-positive rate). This is the price we must now pay for a simple test to detect colorectal cancer.

The clinical problems producing these false-positive results include diverticulosis, adenomatous polyps, and other benign conditions such as hemorrhoids or aspirin-induced bleeding. The analytic problems include detection of red meat fibers in some systems. Pretest rehydration (in Hemoccult II, for example) increases sensitivity, but causes an unacceptable increase in false-positive results.

False-negative test results can occur because of reduced dietary bulk, because of vitamin C ingestion, or because a specimen has not been tested within two to four days of its collection.

REFERENCE
1. Branch WT, Vineyard G: Colorectal carcinoma, in Branch WT (ed): *Office Practice of Medicine*. Philadelphia, WB Saunders, 1982.

□ Clinical Problem

THERAPEUTIC DRUG MONITORING

- An asthmatic patient who has been taking theophylline requires an intravenous (IV) dose. It must be carefully calculated in order to be effective but not toxic.
- An elderly patient has been taking digoxin for cardiac arrhythmia. Is the continuing arrhythmia due to insufficient dosage or to toxicity?
- A patient's epilepsy continues to be out of control. Has the patient really been taking the medication?

Conditions to be identified

- Therapeutic drug levels.
- Toxic drug levels.
- Patient noncompliance.
- Present level of medication to guide dose adjustment.

Basis of laboratory diagnosis

It is now possible to measure therapeutic drug levels in the office lab with a variety of immunochemical techniques. Such testing differs from other laboratory measurements in several respects. The concentrations of most body constituents maintain a relatively stable level during the day, subject to minor circadian variations, but drugs are episodically ingested and subsequently disappear from the blood over time. Interpreting blood drug concentrations depends on knowing when the last dose was taken in relation to when the specimen was collected. The disappearance rate is influenced by uptake into other body compartments, metabolism, and excretion.

Clinically useful interpretation of serum drug levels may depend on appropriate sampling at a certain time after administering the drug (Figure 5-4). Interpreting serum drug levels will also depend on sampling after reaching a steady-state concentration; that is, after a stable dose has been given for a defined period of time (Figure 5-5 and Table 5-1).[1]

A major problem in therapeutic drug monitoring (TDM) is that therapeutic and toxic drug levels are less well defined than are the reference ranges for physiologic blood constituents (Ta-

Steady-state blood digoxin concentrations

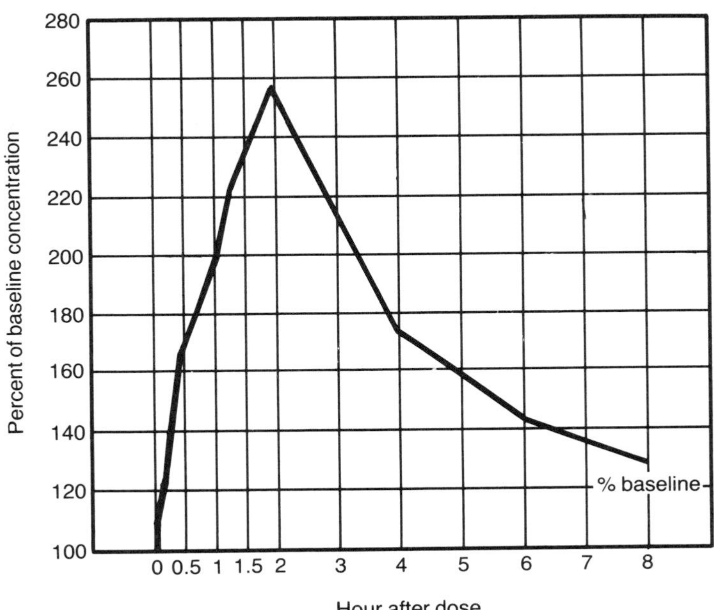

Because of patient-to-patient variation, it's impossible to predict individual response when expressing steady-state concentration as a percentage of the baseline concentration. The data shown are mean values derived from studies of six patients.[3]

ble 5-2).[2] In addition, therapeutic and toxic ranges for some drugs are markedly influenced by the degree of serum protein binding. For others, it may be necessary to measure active metabolites as well as the parent compound.

History, physical examination, and previous laboratory tests

History—particularly finding similar problems in the past—is important in evaluating the patient with suspected digoxin intoxication or the epileptic patient who may not be regularly taking prescribed medication. For example, someone with a history of hypokalemia or fibrillation episodes with digoxin levels consistently in the therapeutic range would be evaluated quite differently from an asymptomatic patient whose digoxin concentration

Blood concentrations after starting oral dosage

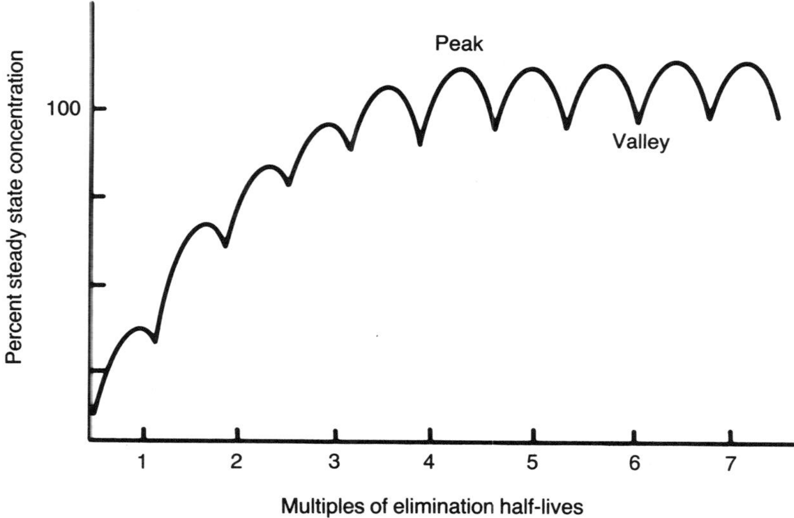

Blood concentrations following initiation of oral dosage of a drug. The maximal steady state concentration of the drug in the blood is not reached until five half lives after starting the medication.

---

was always in the borderline-toxic range. Similarly, the epileptic patient whose previous phenytoin concentrations were highly variable should be followed differently from another whose control was good and whose phenytoin concentrations were stable.

Initial evaluation

As noted earlier, a drug history focusing on potentially allergic or toxic reactions is essential to evaluate these problems. Once drug monitoring is deemed necessary, it will be important to determine exactly when to draw specimens relative to the time of drug administration. It is difficult or impossible to evaluate the drug monitoring value if the specimen is taken at the wrong time in relation to the start of therapy or the last drug dose.

Since drugs are metabolized or excreted at variable rates, correction factors to "normalize" a value taken at the wrong time do not work. A digoxin concentration obtained less than six hours after the previous dose cannot be reliably evaluated. The serum drug level will indicate only whether or not the last dose was actually taken.

Some drugs have very long disappearance times. Phenytoin, for example, has a half-life of 12 to 36 hours. In the case of this drug and others with long half-lives, the time of sampling is less critical. But after changing or starting dosage, it will take longer to use the blood drug level to predict therapeutic effect.

Evaluating potential drug toxicity may require measuring compounds other than the serum drug concentration. A serum potassium assay should be done, for example, if digoxin toxicity is suspected because both factors are synergistic. That is, a low serum potassium will accentuate the toxic effects of an elevated digoxin level. In a patient with no available history or laboratory results, a serum albumin assay may be useful in analyzing phenytoin levels because this drug binds to serum proteins (Table 5-3).

TABLE 5-1

Recommended time for collecting TDM specimens[1]

Drug	Sampling time	Elimination half-life (hours)	Approximate time to reach steady state after dosage change
Carbamazepine	Before next dose	15-30	6 days
Digoxin	6 hours after dose to before the next dose	40	7 days*
Ethosuximide	Before next dose	30-60	5 days(children) 8 days(adults)
Gentamicin	1/2 hour after IV (peak) Before next dose (trough)	2-3	1 day
Phenobarbital	Before next dose	60-90	18 days
Phenytoin	Before next dose	20-30	5 days
Procainamide	1 hour after dose (peak) Before next dose (trough)	3-6	1 day*
Quinidine	1 hour after dose (peak) Before next dose (trough)	6-8	2 days*

*Steady state is achieved sooner with a loading dose.

Suggested therapeutic blood levels of commonly monitored drugs.[2]

Drug	Therapeutic interval
Amikacin	20-30 µg/mL (peak)
	1-8 µg/mL (trough)
Carbamazepine	4-12 µg/mL
Digoxin	0.9-2.0 µg/mL
Disopyramide	2.5-5.0 µg/mL
Ethosuximide	50-100 µg/mL
Gentamicin	6-10 µg/mL
Kanamycin	20-30 µg/mL (peak)
	1-8 µg/mL (trough)
Lidocaine	1.5-5.0 µg/mL
Lithium	0.5-1.2 mmol/L
Phenobarbital	15-40 µg/mL
Phenytoin	10-20 µg/mL
Primidone	5-12 µg/mL
Procainamide	4-10 µg/mL
Procainamide + NAPA	10-30 µg/mL
Quinidine	2-5 µg/mL
Salicylate	150-300 µg/mL
Theophylline	10-20 µg/mL
Tobramycin	6-10 µg/mL
Valproic acid	50-100 µg/mL

Follow-up and management tests

Once the initial drug assay has been performed and a dosage adjustment made, follow-up testing may be important. With theophylline, the object is to choose an effective dose while avoiding toxicity. Repeat measurements of its concentration can be important in determining the most effective dose.

In reducing the dose in suspected digoxin toxicity, monitoring clinical effects of the reduction is the most useful guide.

In the epileptic patient, periodic measurements of phenytoin concentration may help to adjust the dose or to persuade the patient to take the medication regularly. Repeat measurements should not be done too frequently because of the drug's long half-life.

TABLE 5-3

Drugs with more than 80% serum protein binding

Amitriptyline	Lidocaine	Salicylate
Carbamazepine	Nortriptyline	Valproic acid
Desiprimine	Phenytoin	
Imiprimine	Quinidine	

TABLE 5-4

Estimating theophylline dose: A simple approach to using the drug in acutely asthmatic adults with known baseline serum theophylline concentration (STC)

1. Should theophylline be used?
   a) If STC < 20, yes (go to step 2)
   b) If STC > 25, no
   c) If STC >20, < 25, input other factors

2. Should a loading dose be used?
   a) If STC < 12, yes (calculate loading dose; go to step 3)
   b) If STC > 18, no (go to step 3)
   c) If STC >12, < 18, input other factors

3. Should a maintenance infusion be started?
   a) If STC > 20, no
   b) If STC < 15, yes
   c) If STC >15, < 20, input other factors

Note: Theophylline concentrations are given in μg/mL.

Pitfalls of test interpretation

Measuring the drug's blood concentration is but an indirect measurement of its effect at the organ receptor site. As we mentioned, blood concentration and its interpretation are markedly affected by the time of sampling so it's extremely important to obtain the blood sample at the appropriate time. In the case of theophylline, interpretation is based on peak concentration (Table 5-4), so it's impossible to find out whether the dosage causes toxicity if sampling is done after the peak has been reached. Also, most patients now receive sustained-action formulations where the drug is released over a prolonged period. This minimizes the variation between peak and trough concentrations.

Our estimates of therapeutic and toxic concentrations are inexact, but gross variations from the expected concentrations generally indicate whether the patient is receiving too much or too little drug. Variations close to the toxic-therapeutic borderline must be interpreted with caution. This is especially true for serum digoxin levels as its metabolites do have varying degrees of activity that some methods measure.

Hypoalbuminemia results in a larger proportion of the drug in a biologically active, free, or unbound state. Hypoalbuminemic patients taking highly protein-bound drugs such as phenytoin will have a greater drug effect, and thus will require lower dosage than will patients who have a normal albumin level.

REFERENCES

1. Baer DM, Dito WR: *Interpretations in Therapeutic Drug Monitoring.* Chicago, American Society of Clinical Pathologists, 1981.

2. Statland BE: *Clinical Decision Levels for Lab Tests.* Oradell, NJ, Medical Economics Books, 1983.

3. Walsh FM, Sode J: Significance of non-steady-state serum digoxin concentrations. *Am J Clin Pathol* 1975;63:446-450.

☐ Clinical Problem

THYROID TESTING

- A patient with weight *gain,* fatigue, depression, or a change in sleep habits.
- A patient with weight *loss,* fatigue, depression, nervousness, agitation, or a change in sleep habits.

Conditions to be identified

- Hypothyroidism.
- Hyperthyroidism.

Degree of urgency

These disorders usually develop insidiously and do not pose an immediate danger unless other factors, such as scheduled surgery, intervene.

Basis of the laboratory diagnosis

Diagnosis is most commonly based on measuring hormones in the thyroid-pituitary axis. Screening for abnormal thyroid function in symptomatic patients can be done with a serum thyroxine (T_4) determination. Even better is a free T_4 (FT_4). Because most thyroid hormone is bound to specific transport globulins that are subject to modulation by a variety of factors, abnormal T_4 results should be followed with further testing.

If the T_4 is low, determining the thyroid stimulating hormone (TSH) concentration will differentiate hypothyroidism from a variety of conditions that reduce the thyroid transport globulin concentration or functional capacity. If total T_4 is high, FT_4 should be measured. This value will discriminate between hyperthyroidism and those conditions that increase the thyroid binding globulin (TBG) concentration. These few tests are enough to classify most patients with thyroid problems.

Then, if the diagnosis is still in doubt, rather than doing any more tests, the office-based, primary-care physician should probably consult with an endocrinologist about further evaluation. Triiodothyronine (T_3) and free T_3 are not usually necessary in assessing thyroid function.

History, physical examination, and previous lab results

Because onset is insidious, dating it as closely as possible is important. This often involves asking indirectly about changes in behavior, energy, menses, and other functions known to be affected by thyroid dynamics. It can also be helpful to find out whether family members or other independent observers noted a goiter or fullness in the neck.

Physical examination can be particularly helpful in differentiating between hyperthyroidism and hypothyroidism. It is usually possible to detect excessive movements and, if the individual has been seen before, whether such activity is a change. A goiter, especially with an audible bruit, also suggests thyroid dysfunction. Delayed deep tendon reflexes, particularly in a young person, can suggest thyroid dysfunction as can changes in the skin, nails, hair, and eyebrows.

Initial evaluation

When considering the possibility of thyroid dysfunction, the best first test is an FT_4 determination. If this is not readily available, total T_4 is an acceptable substitute, but because of the way serum thyroid transport globulins affect this determination, additional testing will often be required. The free thyroxine index (FTI) can be helpful in clarifying the total T_4 value as a result of variable thyroid transport globulin concentration.

Follow-up and management tests

When the FT_4 determination is abnormally low, the patient is presumed to be hypothyroid. Conversely, someone with a high result is suspected to be hyperthyroid. But before initiating therapy, try to confirm the diagnosis and identify the cause. For example, an elevated TSH confirms primary hypothyroidism. A radioiodine uptake can confirm thyroid dysfunction leading to hyperthyroidism; low uptake will also identify factitious hyperthyroidism in patients surreptitiously taking exogenous thyroid hormone. A thyroid scan is unnecessary under these circumstances unless the clinician wants to evaluate the functional status of an abnormality in the thyroid gland itself—a possible nodule, for example.

If the total T_4 determination is abnormal, the free T_4 could still be within the accepted reference range. Thus, to find out whether the problem is caused by thyroid gland dynamics or by a change in TBG concentration or functional capacity, you should do an FT_4 determination to make the distinction. This will conpensate for changes in total T_4 as a result of changes in TBG concentration or capacity. A resin T_3 uptake test, although less satisfactory, can also be used to derive an FTI. Once an abnormality in the concentration of free thyroxine is confirmed, the next step is to determine the cause of the disorder.

Pitfalls in test interpretation

As we noted, major problems in assessing thyroxine abnormalities center on nonthyroid conditions that modulate the thyroid transport globulins. A common finding is that of elevated female sex steroids (including oral contraceptives and elevated levels during pregnancy), which raise TBG concentration while male hormones, endogenous and exogenous, have the opposite effect. A less well-appreciated fact is the effect of some drugs (phenytoin and high doses of aspirin) in reducing available binding sites on the T_4 transport globulins.

In assessing thyroid gland dynamics, it is also important to consider factitious hyperthyroidism in individuals who are either preoccupied with losing weight or have some connection with the health-care system. Although iodine no longer interferes with thyroid function tests as it once did, it can be the basis for hypothyroidism, particularly in patients with a damaged thyroid gland from surgery or radioiodine therapy.

Finally, although the overwhelming majority of thyroid problems can be diagnosed using this approach, some conditions may escape discovery. Since the laboratory evaluation beyond this point becomes quite complex, it is prudent for the clinician who does not have wide experience in evaluating difficult thyroid problems to consult an endocrinologist.

REFERENCES

1. Howanitz JH, Howanitz PJ: Evaluation of endocrine function, in Henry JB (ed), *Clinical Diagnosis and Management by Laboratory Methods*, ed 17. Philadelphia, WB Saunders, 1984.

2. Larsen PR: Thyroid diseases, in Branch WT (ed), *Office Practice of Medicine*. Philadelphia, WB Saunders, 1982.

☐ Clinical Problem

UNEXPECTED ABNORMAL RESULTS

A patient has an unexpected abnormal result in preadmission testing, multitest screening, or an unrequested test produced by a multichannel profile analyzer.

Conditions to be identified

It is incumbent on the clinician to evaluate unexpected abnormal results to distinguish between those indicating new, significant medical problems and those that are a consequence of how a reference range is defined (Chapter 4). We will discuss unexpected abnormal results in the following analytes:

- Alkaline phosphatase (ALP)
- Bilirubin
- Calcium
- Glucose

- Cholesterol
- Lactate dehydrogenase (LD, LDH)
- Aspartate aminotransferase (AST, SGOT)
- Blood urea nitrogen (BUN)
- Uric acid
- Hematocrit (or hemoglobin)
- Albumin and total protein

Elevated serum ALP activity

Reference values for serum enzyme activity vary with the substrate used, the temperature at which the analysis is performed, and the reagent's formulation. For this discussion, we will use an ALP reference interval of 35 to 120 U/L for adults. To the extent that a particular reference interval differs from this one, the decision level for taking action should change accordingly. Because of a high false-positive rate using this reference range, only ALP elevations greater than 125% of the upper limit (150 U/L in this case) should be evaluated further. Among the clinical causes of increased ALP activity are these:

- Intrahepatic cholestasis because of an infiltrating carcinoma, leukemia, tuberculosis, sarcoidosis amyloidosis, or fibrosis in the liver.
- Extrahepatic cholestasis because of a stone in the common bile duct, a neoplasm retarding normal bile flow, or biliary atresia.
- An increase in osteoblastic activity because of a malignancy that metastacized to bone or because of hyperparathyroidism, either primary or secondary to such problems as vitamin D deficiency or incipient renal failure.
- An ALP-producing tumor.
- Pregnancy.

When ALP values are greater than 125% of the upper reference limit, several procedures are used for further evaluation. Finding elevated serum gamma-glutamyltransferase (GGT) activity often confirms a hepatic problem. But this test (GGT) is very sensitive to small amounts of many hepatic toxins, including alcohol, so it has a high false-positive rate in diagnosing hepatobiliary disease. A normal GGT might indicate a nonhepatic problem such as increased osteoblastic activity, which might be defined with radiologic studies. An increased BUN may indicate renal insufficiency with associated secondary hyperparathyroidism. An increased serum calcium concentration suggests the possibility of primary hyperparathyroidism; a low serum calcium is consistent with secondary hyperparathyroidism. In women of childbearing age, pregnancy should always be considered as a cause of increased ALP activity.

Among the pitfalls in evaluating increased ALP levels is that they are often found with no associated definable clinical problem. Postmenopausal women often have very high ALP values that defy definition, for example, but a diagnostic trial of vitamin D should be considered before abandoning the evaluation.

Continued assessment of the patient, including laboratory studies, over a three- to six-month period may define an underlying malignancy as the cause of increased ALP activity. It must be appreciated, however, that the abnormal value may remain an isolated finding that will persist for years without manifesting a serious medical problem.

Elevated bilirubin

A bilirubin concentration of more than 1.4 mg/dL (the reference range is 0.1 to 1.2 mg/dL in most laboratories) suggests the need for further evaluation. Causes of increased values in adults include these possibilities:

- Extrahepatic biliary obstruction
- Gilbert's disease
- Hemolysis
- Hepatic insufficiency
- Neonatal transient hyperbilirubinemia

Additional testing in adults should include AST, ALP, and prothrombin time. An abnormality in any of these strongly suggests hepatic disease. An elevated serum bilirubin with a normal AST is consistent with Gilbert's disease. Intravascular hemolysis can be confirmed by finding a reduced serum haptoglobin concentration.

Pitfalls in evaluating an elevated bilirubin concentration include both physiologic and methodologic problems. The serum bilirubin concentration may be increased up to 200% in persons who have been fasting for more than 48 hours (Chapter 3). Prolonged tourniquet application during specimen collection can also cause significantly increased bilirubin results.

Elevated serum calcium

Ambulatory patients tend to have higher serum calcium values than do hospitalized, supine patients (reference range: 9.0 to 10.6 mg/dL). Since a large portion of serum calcium is bound to serum albumin, patients with a low albumin reading can also be expected to have a low calcium value. Among the causes of increased serum calcium concentration are these:

- Hyperparathyroidism
- Metastatic carcinoma
- Multiple myeloma
- Sarcoidosis
- Thiazide diuretics (possibly because of otherwise asymptomatic hyperparathyroidism)
- Thyrotoxicosis

A marginally abnormal serum calcium (between 10.6 and 11.0 mg/dL) should be repeated two or three times before doing further studies. But very high serum calcium concentrations may require immediate hospitalization; a value greater than 13.5 mg/dL can be associated with serious, potentially life-threatening arrhythmias. Persistently elevated values between 10.6 and 11.0 mg/dL or a single value of more than 11.0 mg/dL suggests the need for further evaluation that should include repeat serum calcium (in the case of the value above 11.0 mg/dL) and serum albumin, phosphorus, and ALP determinations.

In patients with persistent calcium elevations unassociated with serum protein abnormalities, a parathyroid hormone assay (PTH) can help differentiate hypercalcemia associated with parathyroid suppression (usually from metastatic malignancy) and that caused by overactivity (primary hyperparathyroidism). It is important to remember that PTH values must be interpreted in conjunction with the serum calcium concentration in a specimen drawn at the same time. A "normal" PTH result with a high serum calcium must be considered an abnormal result because an elevated calcium should suppress parathyroid secretion.

Pitfalls in interpreting an unexpectedly abnormal serum calcium result involve both analytic problems and preanalytic sources of variation. One technical consideration is that most chemistry analyzers produce a predictable increase in the calcium values (compared with the true, accurate value, as we discuss in Chapter 13), with the largest increases often seen in the highest values. For this reason, an ionized or free calcium determination may be more accurate in questionable cases.

Preanalytic sources of inaccuracy in serum calcium determinations include prolonged tourniquet application during phlebotomy and the patient's posture before specimen collection.

Elevated serum glucose

The most frequently seen causes of increased serum glucose values are these:
- Chronic renal failure
- Diabetes mellitus
  Maturity-onset (adult)
  Growth-onset (juvenile)
- Other endocrine disorders such as acromegaly, Cushing's syndrome, thyrotoxicosis, and pheochromocytoma
- Pancreatitis
- Physical or emotional stress
- Postprandial glucose testing
- Such medications as corticosteroids, thiazide diuretics, and oral contraceptives

Someone with a fasting blood glucose of 140 mg/dL or greater or a random finding greater than 200 mg/dL should be evaluated further. The obvious pitfalls in evaluating an elevated serum glucose are that the patient may not have fasted before the specimen was collected or may be taking medication that causes elevated values.

Decreased serum glucose

Several conditions can cause low glucose values:
- Adrenocortical insufficiency
- Alimentary hypoglycemia
- Ethanol abuse
- Extrapancreatic neoplasms
- Hypopituitarism
- Insulinoma
- Massive liver disease
- Neonatal glycogen storage disease (Type I)
- Reactive hypoglycemia
- Such medications as insulin, phenformin, sulfonylureas, or salicylates

A serum glucose concentration of less than 45 mg/dL following a 12-hour fast is consistent with but not diagnostic of hypoglycemia. Such values are often associated with anxiety, shakiness, sweating, trembling, and weakness. Headache, irritability, and lethargy may predominate if the hypoglycemic reaction has come on slowly.

Appropriate studies should be done to identify the cause of the hypoglycemia. A five-hour glucose tolerance test might confirm reactive and alimentary hypoglycemia, but diagnosing an insulinoma may require far more extensive studies starting with simultaneous serum glucose and insulin determinations after a 72-hour fast. Immediate therapeutic measures, with deferral of the diagnostic evaluation, should be considered in the case of anyone found to be severely hypoglycemic.

Pitfalls in evaluating a depressed serum glucose value involve clinical and analytic considerations. Delay in the separating of the serum from the cells or in processing the test can cause an artifactually low result. Clinical points to remember are that some individuals, particularly women, develop serum glucose values of less than 45 mg/dL because of prolonged fasting (48 to 72 hours). An especially perplexing problem can be differentiating factitious hypoglycemia and an insulinoma in patients who show significant hypoglycemia (less than 30 mg/dL) during or at the end of a 72-hour fast. Factitious hypoglycemia should be suspected if the patient works in the health care system or possibly has access to insulin through a friend of relative. A useful aid in distinguishing the two forms of hypoglycemia is to determine C-peptide concentration. This is the peptide link that is cleaved and secreted during insulin secretion but is chemically different from therapeutic insulin preparations.

Elevated serum cholesterol

Cholesterol reference values are very age and sex dependent. For our purposes, we will assume a reference interval of 150 to 300 mg/dL.

The most common causes of increased serum cholesterol:
- Biliary obstruction
- Familial (hereditary) hypercholesterolemia
- Hypothyroidism
- Nephrotic syndrome
- Pregnancy

A serum cholesterol concentration greater than 300 mg/dL in an adult indicates a significant risk for atherosclerotic cardiovascular disease. Some authorities strongly argue that cholesterol levels in the upper half of the reference range (220 to 290 mg/dL) suggest an increased risk of disease. Determining high-density lipoprotein cholesterol concentration can help assess this risk, and you may then want to counsel the patient about the roles of exercise, stress, diet, and smoking in minimizing the risk of atherosclerotic disease. The routine use of lipoprotein electrophoresis for these patients is not warranted unless there are coexistant serum triglyceride abnormalities. Most abnormalities can be adequately characterized by measuring cholesterol and triglyceride and watching the refrigerated serum sample for a fatty layer.

Elevated LD activity

Increased serum LD (LDH) concentrations activity may indicate several kinds of disorders:
- Delirium tremens
- Hemolytic disease such as megaloblastic anemia and sickle cell anemia
- Hepatic disorders
- Infectious mononucleosis
- Malignancy including leukemia, lymphoma, and metastatic carcinoma
- Myocardial infarction
- Pulmonary infarction
- Progressive muscular dystrophy
- Trauma

A serum LD finding greater than 300 U/L (reference range: 60 to 220 U/L when the lactate to pyruvate reaction is used at 37 C) suggests the need for additional testing. First, do a repeat LD. If the abnormality is confirmed, further testing should include AST, ALP, and creatine kinase (CK) activity. These markers along with the LD isoenzyme pattern are useful in identifying the source of the increased LD. The following patterns are of interest:
- An increase in LD 1 can be associated with cardiac damage or the listed RBC disorders.
- An increase in LD 2, 3, or 4 is associated with malignancy, pulmonary disease, or renal disease.

- An increase in LD 5 is often associated with liver
  disease or skeletal muscle disorders.

Isolated LD increases are often seen in routine chemical profiles. Repeat tests usually obviate the need for further evaluation since their results often return to the reference interval. Some older patients with an unexpected LD elevation may in fact have incipient pernicious anemia that might respond to a therapeutic trial of vitamin B_{12}, causing reticulocytosis and a return to the reference range.

Elevated AST activity

Among the causes of increased AST (SGOT) values are the following diseases:

- Hepatocellular destruction, as in viral, toxic, or
  alcoholic hepatitis
- In vivo hemolysis
- Musculoskeletal disease
- Myocardial infarction
- Posthepatic obstructive biliary tract disease
- Pulmonary infarction

A serum AST value greater than 60 U/L (reference range: 8 to 40 U/L when the reaction is measured at 37 C) suggests the need for further evaluation. Helpful tests include serum alanine aminotransferase (ALT, formerly called SGPT), CK, ALP, and bilirubin.

Potential pitfalls in evaluating the elevated AST can be the definition of normality (statistical outliers) and recent ingestion of ethanol or other hepatotoxic drugs. Consequently, if the AST is between 40 and 60 U/L, further evaluation is generally not recommended unless there is reason to suspect hepatitis. If hepatitis B infection is a reasonable possibility, then test for its surface antigen.

Elevated BUN

The following conditions, the most important of which is renal insufficiency, may cause increased serum BUN values:

- Dehydration
- Gastrointestinal (GI) bleeding
- High-protein diet
- Impaired renal function
- Postrenal azotemia

- Prerenal azotemia, as seen in congestive heart
  failure or shock
- Such drugs as corticosteroids and tetracycline

Further evaluation of an increased BUN should include a creatinine determination. Increases in both these analytes suggest renal impairment; an increase in BUN and a normal serum creatinine suggest prerenal azotemia.

Potential pitfalls in interpreting an elevated BUN include nonpathologic dehydration or an unknown high-protein diet.

Elevation of uric acid

Among the causes of increased uric acid are the following:
- Chronic lead nephropathy
- Diet (high protein or high nucleoprotein)
- Gout
- Ketoacidosis
- Lactate excess, as after ethanol ingestion
- Leukemia, lymphoma, or polycythemia vera
- Polycystic kidneys
- Renal failure
- Such antiuricosuric drugs as diuretics

A uric acid level greater than 8.0 mg/dL (reference range: 2.5 to 7.0 mg/dL) suggests the need for further evaluation. Values greater than 10.7 mg/dL indicate an increased risk of developing renal calculi or joint tophi.

A potential problem in determining the cause of an elevated uric acid level is that the patient has not disclosed a high protein diet (actually high protein and high nucleoprotein) or recent ethanol ingestion with a consequent increase in serum urates.

Decreased hematocrit

A hematocrit of less than 36% in men or 30% in women (or a hemoglobin of 12 or 10 gm/dL, respectively) requires further evaluation to determine the cause of the anemia.

The causes of decreased hematocrit values or hemoglobin concentration can be divided into problems associated with the number—either increased or decreased—of circulating reticulocytes. An increase is seen with hemolytic anemias (as from immunologic causes) and those caused by trauma to red cells, abnormalities of the RBC membrane, hemoglobinopathies, or red cell enzyme deficiencies. A decreased or normal value in circulating reticulocytes is associated with hypochromic microcytic anemia (iron deficiency, thalassemia, anemia of chronic disease, sideroblastic anemia), macrocytic anemia (deficiency of vitamin B_{12} or folate or as a consequence of some chemotherapeutic agents), and normochromic anemia (bone marrow depression or failure).

To the trained eye, the red cell smear can be quite helpful in clarifying the differential diagnosis of anemia. Smaller RBCs on the smear (decreased mean corpuscular volume, MCV) suggests iron deficiency anemia, while large cells suggest folate or B_{12} deficiency. These causes can be confirmed by determining the serum iron, iron binding capacity, and ferritin in the former case and the serum B_{12} and folate in the latter.

Abnormalities in serum albumin and total protein

Total protein in healthy adult serum is 6 to 8 g/dL. The reference interval for albumin is 3.5 to 5.0 g/dL. Among the causes for decreased albumin are these:

- Acute and chronic inflammation
- Extensive burns
- Liver insufficiency with decreased albumin synthesis
- Malignancy
- Pregnancy
- Renal disease, such as the nephrotic syndrome with urinary protein loss
- Severe malnutrition

An increase in total protein concentration may be caused by the following conditions:

- Chronic inflammation
- Dehydration
- Multiple myeloma (IgG, IgA)
- Sarcoidosis

A combined increase in total protein concentration and decrease in albumin is highly suggestive of multiple myeloma. The next step is to determine the electrophoretic pattern of serum and urine proteins; if an abnormal protein pattern is found in either, assays for specific classes of immunoglobulin (by immuno-electrophoresis or immunoprecipitation techniques) can be very helpful in confirming the diagnosis of multiple myeloma and, to some extent, in determining therapy and estimating prognosis.

A decrease in the albumin/globulin ratio is often seen in liver disease. The synthesis of albumin is decreased while the concentration of immunoglobulins accounts for the increase in the globulin fraction.

☐ Clinical Problem

URINARY TRACT INFECTION

Dysuria and frequency in a young woman.

Conditions to be identified

Upper or lower urinary tract infection.

Degree of urgency

Although most untreated urinary tract infections (UTIs) are not dangerous, patients usually see them as urgent problems because of the discomfort they cause. Concern about an upper tract infection is increased if the patient is febrile or has lumbar or costovertebral pain.

Basis of the laboratory diagnosis

Urine culture is the definitive method for diagnosing UTI, but because of the time it takes to get a result and because of the patient's discomfort, a number of other approaches have been developed to speed the diagnosis. A Gram stain of fresh unspun urine can be of value if organisms can be identified. Requiring less skill on the part of the operator are nitrite strips that detect the presence of nonfermenting gram-negative bacteria in urine. Bacteriologic approaches other than culture can identify the most common urinary pathogens, but not all of them.

Chemical and microscopic analyses are also used to diagnose UTIs. One classic method is to look for granulocytes and granulocyte casts in centrifuged urine sediment. This test is widely used, but because of the many interfering substances in sediment, it requires considerable skill and training to get meaningful results. Both preparing and examining the sediment are time-consuming, making the test labor intensive and costly.

In the ambulatory-care setting, several approaches have been used to maximize the time spent looking for sediments with positive findings. One of these is to screen for urinary protein, glucose, or blood with a chemical test, and do further microscopic testing only on positive results. This reduces the labor involved by a factor of five to 10 without significantly reducing clinical utility.

Another approach is to use a chemical test for urinary esterases. Neutrophilic granulocytes contain many esterases that catalyze the hydrolysis of an ester to produce its alcohol and acid; other RBCs and cells from the urinary tract do not contain these proteins. The reagent strip screens for granulocytes and can thus select the specimens with a higher probability of growing a positive culture. Such nonculture methods are an indirect—and thus less accurate—way to diagnose UTIs, but their results are much faster and are effective for guiding therapy.

Most lower UTIs in women resolve spontaneously with no long-standing kidney damage. Accordingly one therapeutic approach is to give a single large antibiotic dose at the initial evaluation to patients who have no symptoms or indications of upper tract infection, such as costovertebral angle tenderness, or UTI within the past six months. Patients who respond to this approach (a large majority) are considered to have had an uncomplicated lower tract infection; those who do not are presumed to have an upper tract infection and are given an additional course of antibiotics.

History, physical examination, and previous lab results

Documenting previous UTIs can be very helpful in the diagnostic process, particularly if the circumstances of the current episode are similar to those in the past (for example, following sexual intercourse). It is also important to ascertain whether the patient has had a UTI during the past six months. If so, it would argue against the therapeutic trial approach just described and suggest that a urine specimen for culture and susceptibility should be obtained before starting therapy. As most clinicians appreciate, differentiating a UTI from urethral irritation as a result of a vaginal discharge can be difficult with antibiotic therapy potentially aggravating the latter condition by increasing the risk of a yeast infection.

Initial evaluation

The diagnosis of UTI is classically confirmed with a urine culture taken before the start of therapy. Since the results of this test are not available for at least 24 to 48 hours, the office laboratory may use leukocyte esterase urine test strips instead of or in addition to the urine culture. We do not recommend the use of nitrite reagent strips in the office setting although patients with recurrent UTIs may use them to monitor an increase in the concentration of urinary microorganisms. Alternatively, the therapeutic trial approach can be used with patients selected using the criteria described before.

Follow-up and management tests

In patients with their first uncomplicated UTI during a six-month period, no further diagnostic or management tests are indicated. But if the patient has had an earlier UTI, it is best to perform antibiotic susceptibility testing of any isolates. Most authorities do not recommend reculturing the urine after the course of antibiotics, but suggest waiting to see if symptoms develop again for further evaluation.

Pitfalls in test interpretation

The threshold for diagnosing UTI in a young, otherwise healthy woman is based on finding more than 100,000 colonies of a pathogen in the urine culture. As with other bacteriologic diagnoses, the prerequisite for accurate diagnosis is a properly collected specimen, and this is particularly important in evaluating urine (Chapter 3 outlines the protocol for collecting a clean-voided specimen).

The other major pitfall in diagnosing UTIs is a result of the frequency with which some women get these infections and the discomfort they cause. Women who think they are developing an infection often use antibiotics from a previous episode before seeking medical assistance, which often means a negative culture in spite of an actual UTI.

Although the nonbacteriologic methods of diagnosing UTI are less sensitive than the bacteriologic approach, which is the definitive reference method, they can be operationally effective in guiding therapy. It is important, however, to understand the limitations of the methodology and to be prepared to reconsider the diagnosis if the patient does not respond to therapy.

REFERENCES

1. Bradley M, Schumann GB: Examination of urine, in Henry JB (ed), *Clinical Diagnosis and Management by Laboratory Methods*, ed 17. Philadelphia, WB Saunders, 1984.

2. Branch WT: Urinary tract infections, in Branch WT (ed), *Office Practice of Medicine*. Philadelphia, WB Saunders, 1982.

3. Washington JA: Medical bacteriology, in Henry JB (ed), *Clinical Diagnosis and Management by Laboratory Methods*, ed 17. Philadelphia, WB Saunders, 1984.

□ Clinical Problem

WEIGHT LOSS

A 62-year-old man whose chief complaint is weight loss.

Conditions to be identified

A long list of conditions is associated with weight loss (Table 5-5). Some of these will be obvious from the history and physical examination. Other problems for which laboratory testing can be helpful include digoxin toxicity, hypercalcemia, hypokalemia, uremia, diabetes, hyperthyroidism, infection with parasites, and occult malignancy.

Basis of the laboratory diagnosis

Many conditions can cause unplanned weight loss. The laboratory has two major roles: It may confirm or rule out conditions suggested by findings from the patient's history and physical examination, or it may detect changes consistent with a diagnosis that was not evident from those findings.

History, physical examination, and previous laboratory studies

The history and physical examination provide important clues to the cause of weight loss. Helpful in the differential diagnosis are associated symptoms, the duration and extent of the weight loss, any concomitant medical conditions, and the use of medications. It is important to assess whether the history, signs, or symptoms point to decreased nutrient intake, increased nutrient loss, impaired absorption, or an excess demand for nutrients.

Some important causes of weight loss

Decreased caloric intake
Alcoholism
Anorexia nervosa
Anxiety
Chronic congestive heart failure
Chronic inflammatory disease
Depression
Drugs (digoxin toxicity, amphetamines, antitumor agents)
Esophageal disease
Gastrointestinal disease worsened by food
Hypercalcemia
Hypokalemia
Malignancy
Poor dentition
Prodrome of viral hepatitis
Uremia

Increased nutrient loss
Drainage from a fistulous tract
Persistent diarrhea
Recurrent vomiting
Uncontrolled diabetes mellitus

Impaired nutrient absorption
Blind loop syndrome
Cholestasis
Drugs (cholestyramine, cathartics)
Parasitic infection (giardiasis)
Pancreatic insufficiency
Postgastrectomy
Small bowel disease

Excess caloric metabolism
Amphetamine abuse
Emotional states (manic disease)
Fever
Hyperthyroidism
Malignancy

Initial evaluation

The laboratory can be especially useful in investigating weight loss as a result of decreased nutrient intake. Loss of appetite may be associated with drug toxicity (especially from digoxin), hypercalcemia, hypokalemia, uremia, or malignancy. Increased nutritional loss, on the other hand, can result from diabetes mellitus, persistent diarrhea, recurrent vomiting, or occasionally drainage from a fistula tract. Impaired absorption can be associated with biliary obstruction, pancreatic insufficiency, or parasitic infection (such as giardiasis). Weight loss as a result of increased metabolic demand may occur in hyperthyroidism, fever, and malignancy. The initial diagnostic evaluation can, therefore, be firmly based on findings from the history and physical examination, and it can be confirmed by laboratory tests directed toward identification of the high probability disorders.

REFERENCE

1. Goroll AH, May LA, Mulley AG: *Primary Care Medicine. Office Evaluation and Management of the Adult Patient.* Philadelphia, Lippincott, 1981, pp 29-33.

Economics and regulatory foundations

6

Regulation and reimbursement

Reimbursement and regulatory policies have generally encouraged diagnostic testing in physicians' office laboratories. Recent legislative changes, however, have sought to equalize their position vis à vis independent and hospital labs. This chapter discusses some of those changes and provides an up-to-date summary of current regulation of in-office laboratories.

FEDERAL REGULATION

Physicians who do laboratory tests in their own offices are not generally subject to federal regulation if they are testing only their own patients. As long as the tests are an adjunct to treating only their own patients, such laboratories are excluded from licensure requirements of the Clinical Laboratories Improvement Act (CLIA) of 1967 and the 1974 Medicare independent laboratory program, even if specimens are solicited or accepted across state lines and in interstate commerce. The physicians' office laboratory is exempt from CLIA even if it serves a large group of practitioners.

Medicare laboratory regulations, the Conditions for Coverage of Services of Independent Laboratories, are of greater significance than CLIA to an office lab. Generally, if the laboratory performs tests only for the physician's own patients, it is exempt from Medicare regulations governing laboratory operation and performance. But under certain circumstances, a physician's office lab can lose its Medicare exemption. If the lab is "held out" as available to perform testing for other physicians' patients or if it accepts on referral more than 100 specimens a year in any one of six categories—microbiology and serology, chemistry, immuno-hematology, hematology, pathology, or radiobioassay—it is subject to Medicare's comprehensive regulations for independent labs. A group practice or controlled corporate laboratory must meet still other conditions or lose its exemption from Medicare regulations. Eligibility for state Medicaid payments is generally on the same basis as Medicare.

As we said, Medicare's Conditions for Coverage apply to physicians' office laboratories when the laboratories are held out as available for diagnostic testing. This definition is met whenever 1) signs in, on, or near the office indicate the availability of laboratory tests; or 2) the laboratory is listed in the telephone directory. If it is held out for testing, the laboratory is subject to Medicare regulation regardless of the number of specimens it accepts on referral.

Group practice laboratories (for two or more physicians) may also be exempt as a physicians' laboratory under Medicare if they are operated according to the requirements for a solo practitioner. That is, the laboratory must be operated for the group's patients, it must not be held out as available for referral work, and it must not accept more than 100 specimens in any category on referral from physicians outside the group. To assure an exemption, each member of the group should also be jointly identified as an owner or leasee of the laboratory property and premises. Joint responsibility for the laboratory's operating costs is also advisable.

If the laboratory exceeds the 100-specimens-a-year test or is otherwise determined to be nonexempt, it has several alternatives: It can stop accepting referral specimens; it may decide not to seek Medicare reimbursement for referral work; or it can comply with Medicare's Conditions for Coverage. These are a detailed set of performance standards that the lab must meet in such areas as compliance with state laws, qualifications of the laboratory director and other personnel, proficiency testing, the adequacy of records and facilities, and quality control.[1]

When the 98th Congress established a uniform fee schedule for outpatient laboratory testing reimbursed by Medicare, some legislators questioned Medicare's differential performance standards for various laboratories in the face of standardized reimbursement. Medicare sets rigorous performance and personnel standards for hospital and commercial laboratories, but none so far has been promulgated for testing done in private physicians' offices. Reports from Washington, DC, suggested that Congress might want to develop legislation to require standards for office laboratories; if it did, such efforts would undoubtedly meet resistance from organized medicine.

Concern about regulating office laboratories is based on the belief that test results produced in this setting vary significantly more than they do in hospital or independent laboratories. New, superficially simple analytic systems let nonprofessional office staff produce results that can be directly translated into patient management decisions; this development has increased the pressure for regulation to promote quality performance in the office lab. Some states have already undertaken such regulation (Table 6-1).

STATE REGULATION

States are primarily concerned with issues related to quality assurance. Consequently, the regulations are generally concerned with setting standards for personnel, safety, and quality control programs. They often mandate proficiency testing as an objective assessment of the quality of the lab's performance.

In most states, a laboratory operated in relation to a medical practice is exempt from regulatory licensure and performance requirements, but the laws vary widely from state to state. Among the factors most often considered are 1) the number of practitioners operating and using the laboratory facilities; 2) whether testing is done solely for the physician's or the group's own patients; 3) the types of tests performed; and 4) who is actually performing the tests. We will consider four examples of how these factors are applied.

Arizona. Physician-owned and -operated laboratories are exempt from licensure and performance standards when the laboratory is performing tests only for the doctor's patients.

Idaho. A physician's or group practice office laboratory that performs tests for the doctor's own patients is exempt from state regulations only if the physician personally performs the test.

TABLE 6-1

State regulation of physicians' office laboratories

State	MD lab (1)	Exemption: number of doctors (2)	Hospital lab (3)	Survey (4)	Inspection (5)	Personnel rules (6)
Alabama	N		Y	N	N	N
Alaska	N		Y	N	N	N
Arizona	N		Y	N	N	N
Arkansas	N		N	N	N	N
California	N		Y	Y	N	N

Doctors' office labs that accept Medicaid payment must meet all Medicare rules applicable to those labs. All labs, even those exempt from state licensing, must perform proficiency testing.

State	MD lab (1)	Exemption: number of doctors (2)	Hospital lab (3)	Survey (4)	Inspection (5)	Personnel rules (6)
Colorado	N		Y	N	N	N
Connecticut	N		Y	N	N	N

Exempted labs must register annually. New rules covering doctors' office labs are being drafted. Personnel standards and proficiency surveys would be required.

State	MD lab (1)	Exemption: number of doctors (2)	Hospital lab (3)	Survey (4)	Inspection (5)	Personnel rules (6)
Delaware	N		Y	N	N	N

Training and consultation is available to all labs. Proficiency testing in syphilis serology is offered.

State	MD lab (1)	Exemption: number of doctors (2)	Hospital lab (3)	Survey (4)	Inspection (5)	Personnel rules (6)
District of Columbia	N		N	N	N	N

Federal Medicare and CLIA regulations are followed.

State	MD lab (1)	Exemption: number of doctors (2)	Hospital lab (3)	Survey (4)	Inspection (5)	Personnel rules (6)
Florida	Y	<6	Y	Y	Y	Y
Georgia	N		Y	N	N	N
Hawaii	N		Y	Y	Y	N

New regulations are being considered. Proficiency testing can be required of any lab but this has not been done in practice. Some labs have asked for voluntary licensing.

State	MD lab (1)	Exemption: number of doctors (2)	Hospital lab (3)	Survey (4)	Inspection (5)	Personnel rules (6)
Idaho	Y	None	Y	Y	Y	N
Illinois	N		Y	N	N	N
Indiana	N		N	N	N	N
Iowa	N		N	N	N	N
Kansas	N		Y	N	N	N
Kentucky	N		Y	N	N	N
Louisiana	N		N	N	N	N
Maine	N		Y	N	N	N
Maryland	Y	<4	Y	Y	N	N

Proficiency testing is required of all physicians doing laboratory tests regardless of the number of physicians in the group, although some simple lab procedures are exempt from proficiency testing. New regulations will soon require on-site inspection of office labs with four or more physicians in the group.

State	MD lab (1)	Exemption: number of doctors (2)	Hospital lab (3)	Survey (4)	Inspection (5)	Personnel rules (6)
Massachusetts	Y	<3	Y	Y	Y	Y

Requirements are based on amount and complexity of testing.

State	MD lab (1)	Exemption: number of doctors (2)	Hospital lab (3)	Survey (4)	Inspection (5)	Personnel rules (6)
Michigan	Y	<6	Y	Y	Y	Y

The state department of health offers a voluntary proficiency testing program, continuing education, and consultation.

Key: (1) Y = The doctor's office lab is registered or licensed, even if tests are done only on his or her patients and under his or her direction.
    (2) The number of physicians in a group, below which no regulation is in effect.
    (3) Y = Hospital or independent labs are regulated.

State	MD lab (1)	Exemption: number of doctors (2)	Hospital lab (3)	Survey (4)	Inspection (5)	Personnel rules (6)
Mississippi	N		N	N	N	N
Missouri	N		N	N	N	N
Montana	N		Y	N	N	N
Nevada	Y		Y	Y	Y	Y

Proficiency testing and inspection may be required for all labs.

State	MD lab (1)	Exemption: number of doctors (2)	Hospital lab (3)	Survey (4)	Inspection (5)	Personnel rules (6)
New Hampshire	N		Y	Y	N	N

Proficiency testing may be required for all labs.

State	MD lab (1)	Exemption: number of doctors (2)	Hospital lab (3)	Survey (4)	Inspection (5)	Personnel rules (6)
New Jersey	Y	<5	Y	Y	Y	Y

Regulations do not exempt any labs, but now only groups of five or more physicians must license their labs. Regulations are under review and may be revised to include all physicians' office labs.

State	MD lab (1)	Exemption: number of doctors (2)	Hospital lab (3)	Survey (4)	Inspection (5)	Personnel rules (6)
New Mexico	N		N	N	N	N

Training and consultation are available to small labs.

State	MD lab (1)	Exemption: number of doctors (2)	Hospital lab (3)	Survey (4)	Inspection (5)	Personnel rules (6)
New York	N		Y	N	N	N
North Carolina	N		N	N	N	N
North Dakota	N		N	N	N	
Ohio	N		N	N	N	N
Oklahoma	N		N	N	N	N
Oregon	Y	<5	Y	Y	Y	Y
Pennsylvania	Y	None	Y	Y	Y	Y

Requirements for licensing, proficiency testing, inspections, and personnel qualifications are related to the amount and complexity of testing.

State	MD lab (1)	Exemption: number of doctors (2)	Hospital lab (3)	Survey (4)	Inspection (5)	Personnel rules (6)
Puerto Rico	Y		Y	Y	Y	Y
Rhode Island	N		Y	N	N	N
South Carolina	N		N	N	N	N
South Dakota	N		N	N	N	N
Tennessee	N		Y	N	N	N
Texas	N		N	N	N	N
Utah	N		Y	N	N	N

The present law is being reviewed.

State	MD lab (1)	Exemption: number of doctors (2)	Hospital lab (3)	Survey (4)	Inspection (5)	Personnel rules (6)
Vermont	N		Y	N	N	N
Virginia	N		N	N	N	N
Washington	N		Y	N	N	N
West Virginia	N		Y	Y	Y	Y

Only those doctors' office labs accepting Medicaid reimbursement are covered by regulations.

State	MD lab (1)	Exemption: number of doctors (2)	Hospital lab (3)	Survey (4)	Inspection (5)	Personnel rules (6)
Wisconsin	Y	<3	Y	Y	Y	Y
Wyoming	Y	None	Y	Y	Y	Y

Requirements are related to lab complexity. New rules are being drafted.

(4) Y = Proficiency survey is required for regulated doctors' office labs.
(5) Y = On-site inspection is authorized under the state's rules in regulated doctors' office labs.
(6) Y = Law or rules authorize personnel qualifications for director, supervisor, or technician in regulated doctors' office labs.

Delegation of testing to a nurse or office employee brings the lab under state regulation. If the laboratory is under state regulation, it must participate in proficiency surveys and on-site inspections and meet quality-control requirements.

Oregon. Laboratories operated by fewer than five physicians performing tests for their own patients are exempt from state regulation. If five or more physicians are in the group, the laboratory is subject to all the regulatory requirements applicable to independent labs.[2]

California. Until 1984, an individual physician doing tests for his or her own patients was exempt from licensing and performance requirements—although all laboratories were subject to proficiency testing. A new law now requires physicians doing tests for their own patients to meet the same licensing requirements as any other lab in the state if they want to receive MediCal (the state's Medicaid) reimbursement.

California's laboratory licensure requirements also include detailed personnel requirements for clinical laboratory bioanalysts, clinical laboratory or limited technologists, clinical chemists, clinical microbiologists, and trainees. These personnel must be licensed by the state health department. Licensing requires each individual to meet education and experience qualifications, and all but trainees must pass a qualifying examination.

In addition, licensed laboratories in California must maintain quality-control programs acceptable to the health department. They must include keeping records, validating calibration and equipment maintenance, using standards and reference materials, and maintaining procedure manuals. Reagents and stains must be dated and initialed when prepared, or dated when received. If they are commercially prepared, reagents must be dated when opened. Reagents and stains also must be labeled to indicate identity, titer, concentration, recommended storage temperature, expiration data, and other pertinent information.[2] The new law also specifies that when the Department of Health Services contracts for clinical laboratory services, the contractor must be a clinical lab licensed or certified by the state.[3]

Although most states have not yet subjected physician office laboratories to licensure or regulation, 11 have set operating standards for at least some of the office labs in their jurisdiction. The conditions for regulation vary. They are generally based on the number of physicians in the group the lab serves, the complexity of the procedures it performs, or whether the lab does tests for Medicaid patients.

Full regulation for these laboratories usually includes standards for all personnel involved in the testing process (from the bench technologist to the director) and requires a quality assurance program (including preventive equipment maintenance, quality control [QC] of analytic systems to provide early warning of problems, and participation in a proficiency testing program for all analyses processed in the office lab). These very requirements played a significant role in bringing the reliability of information produced by big high-volume laboratories to the level it is today.

Most states do not now regulate laboratories—in physicians' offices or elsewhere—since federal regulations meet their perceived needs. But it seems likely that office laboratories may come under such rules in the near future. They are currently under consideration in Connecticut, Hawaii, Maryland, New Jersey, Utah, and Wyoming. The approaches used by Idaho[4,5] and Pennsylvania (Table 6-2) are likely to provide a direction that many others will find appealing because they establish a framework for assuring quality but at the same time try to minimize the economic burden for both the state and the practitioner.

The important issue to watch as states approach regulation is that of personnel qualifications. The regulations for limited service office labs in both Pennsylvania and Idaho focus on using proficiency testing to evaluate the lab's performance in the context of a required quality-assurance program. They do not specify training or education requirements for office lab personnel—restrictions that would substantially raise the operating cost of an office lab.

REIMBURSEMENT

The Deficit Reduction Act of 1984 brought a major change in Medicare reimbursement for outpatient testing. Before then, payments for covered laboratory services performed by independent laboratories or by physicians in their offices, were made on a reasonable charge basis under Part B of Medicare. The law provided that payment for covered services would be 80% of reasonable charges. For certain services, however, such as commonly ordered laboratory tests, Medicare could limit the reasonable

TABLE 6-2

How Pennsylvania regulates laboratory testing in physicians' office laboratories[9]

Level I. These tests, if performed only on one's patients, require registering the facility with the state health department:
   A. Chemical examination of urine by dipstick or tablet methods for the following constituents: glucose, ketone bodies, urobilinogen, blood, pH, bilirubin;
   B. Chemical examination of blood by dipstick or tablet methods for glucose;
   C. Microscopic examination of urine sediment and specific gravity by a method approved by the health department;
   D. Pregnancy tests;
   E. White cell count;
   F. Hematocrit;
   G. Hemoglobin with a method approved by the department;
   H. Sedimentation rate of blood with a method approved by the department;
   I. Primary culturing for transmittal to a licensed laboratory including any required preincubation;
   J. Qualitative chemical examination of stool for occult blood;
   K. Microscopic examination for pinworms;
   L. Microscopic examination for *Trichomonas vaginalis;*
   M. Sickle cell test for screening purposes only.

Level II. These tests, if performed only on one's own patients now require registration with the state health department plus a $25 fee, successful participation in an approved proficiency testing program (with results released to the department), and adherence to the department's quality-control regulations:
   N. Differential count;
   O. Prothrombin time;
   P. Blood glucose;
   Q. Mononucleosis testing;
   R. Throat cultures for beta strep, including use of bacitracin disks
   S. Screens and colony counts for urinary tract infections. This does not include identification and susceptibility testing.

Level III. If the lab performs any procedures not on the these lists, all the tests it does will be subject to licensure, regular inspection, and successful participation in an approved proficiency testing program.

charge to the lowest charge widely and consistently available in a locality. The local carrier determines this charge.

Another change is that since July 1984, Medicare has reimbursed all outpatient clinical laboratory services according to a fee schedule. This represents the culmination of several events over the previous four years. In 1980, Congress limited a physician's ability to mark up the charge for a laboratory test under both Medicare and Medicaid. When the physician's reimbursement claim identified an outside laboratory and the charge to the physician, the physician's reimbursable charge would be the lesser of 1) the laboratory's reasonable charge for the test, or 2) the actual charge to the physician plus a nominal fee for collecting and handling the specimen. If the physician's reimbursement claim did not identify the outside laboratory or the amount charged, reimbursement was based on the lowest charge available in the locality.

In October 1982, the Health Care Financing Administration (HCFA) convened a task force to examine reimbursement of diagnostic laboratory services. This was in response to considerable attention and criticism of how Medicare Part B and Medicaid were paying for these services. Much of this criticism was leveled at the pricing policies of independent laboratories that charged Medicare and physicians different prices for the same test. Physician's office lab billing was also a target because physicians marked up independent laboratory prices. In February 1984, the task force presented a package of recommendations that included a national fee schedule for Medicare reimbursement of all diagnostic laboratory services.[6]

Congress, in an effort to make a dent in the budget deficit, proposed its own version of a national fee schedule for laboratory services, with an estimated cut of $900 million. It was included in the omnibus Deficit Reduction Act of 1984 and was based on a percentage of prevailing charges for all clinical outpatient diagnostic laboratory services. The fee schedule is carrierwide and covers testing performed in all clinical laboratories although physicians' office and independent laboratories are treated somewhat differently from hospital labs.

The three-year, carrierwide schedule for hospital outpatient services is based on 62% of the prevailing charges for the year beginning July 1, 1984. After the three-year period, reimbursement for hospital outpatient laboratory services would revert to cost reimbursement, unless Congress takes steps to include such services under a national fee schedule. The General Accounting Office (GAO) and HCFA were to study the impact of the fee schedule and report to Congress by June 30, 1985, on the appropriateness of moving to a national fee schedule for hospital laboratories.

The law also made independent and physician's office laboratories initially subject to a transitional, three-year, carrierwide fee schedule at 60% of the prevailing charges for the year beginning July 1, 1984. At the end of three years, these laboratories will come under a national fee schedule, which would be adjusted annually to reflect changes in the Consumer Price Index. The Secretary of Health and Human Services (HHS) may make adjustments or exceptions to the fee schedule to ensure adequate reimbursement for 1) laboratory tests performed during an emergency, 2) certain low-volume, high-cost tests, and 3) technological changes.

Independent and hospital laboratory (outpatient) services are required to accept Medicare assignment. Physicians may now accept assignment on a case-by-case basis. When they accept assignment, reimbursement is at 100% of the fee schedule; when they do not, reimbursement is at 80%, with a 20% coinsurance requirement for beneficiaries.

Direct billing is required, and physicians can bill Medicare only if they (or another physician with whom they share their practice) personally perform or supervise the test. Medicare will also pay $3 to the hospital lab, independent lab, or physician for collecting a specimen. In addition, the HHS Secretary is required to simplify current billing requirements for laboratory services.

FUTURE TRENDS IN REIMBURSEMENT AND REGULATION

We have little hard information on physician's office testing, partly because of a lack of regulatory activity in this area. Market research for manufacturers of laboratory test kits and equipment suggests that as many as 80,000 to 100,000 physicians perform some laboratory tests in their own offices. Some estimates go as high as 190,000 offices. The American Academy of Family Physicians estimates that more than 80% of family physicians include lab work in their offices.[7] The American Society of Internal Medicine estimates that at least 77% of its members do so.

Manufacturers and independent laboratory owners feel that physician's office testing is the most rapidly growing segment of the market. This growth is due, in part, to technological advances that either reduce the size and cost of automated equipment or that replace complex testing methods requiring highly trained personnel with simple-to-use, inexpensive test kits. And not only the number of physicians' office labs but also the volume of testing done is growing. Frost and Sullivan, a New York market research firm, reported that test volume in group practice laboratories doubled between 1976 and 1982, while the number of labs increased by only 3%. There's been some recent speculation that the Medicare fee schedule might dampen this trend, however.

Industry feels that the growth will continue. Prospective payment and diagnosis-related groups (DRGs) force the trend toward ambulatory care. And as hospitals shorten inpatient stays, more preadmission testing and follow-up testing will be done on an outpatient basis.

The fee-schedule incentives are in conflict here. Physicians will have an economic incentive to do some testing in their own offices, because with direct billing they can no longer mark up discounted tests from independent laboratories. They will be reimbursed only for the tests they personally perform or supervise, however.

Reimbursement policy or practice for office testing has not changed very recently, but concern about the economic impact of this technology has continued unabated. As a uniform fee schedule for hospital and independent laboratory testing becomes established, pressure will undoubtedly develop for physician's office labs to receive the same reimbursement. The issues of fair and equal treatment of all laboratories with regard to reimbursement as well as regulation will surely be raised. The Office of Technology Assessment (OTA) has been examining alternative payment methods for clinical laboratory services.

There will also be a strong incentive to perform testing in a cost-effective manner, and some physicians may find they cannot do the test for what Medicare is willing to pay—particularly if the lab becomes regulated. The physician must then weigh the benefits of such testing, both to the patient and to the practice. Medicare is offering fewer billing headaches (100% reimbursement for accepted assignment) and less paperwork but at a reduced fee (60% of the prevailing). It should be kept in perspective, however, that these regulations apply only to testing done on Medicare patients who may be less than 30% of a physician's patient load.

As for the impact of a national fee schedule on third-party reimbursement policy, a lot can be learned from the payers' response to DRGs. Third-party payers are quite concerned about a cost shift as a result of these attempts to cap or lower costs. They are monitoring the DRG system and feel they will be able to show a cost shift. An official policy of the Health Insurance Association of America (HIAA) is that the Federal reimbursement system should be an all-payer system, that is, all insurers including the government should be under the same system. Blue Cross/Blue Shield has responded by actually trying out its own DRG system in at least one state (Kansas). Should the national fee schedule result in a cost shift, insurers will undoubtedly demand an all-payer fee schedule.

A continued trend toward physicians' office testing worries independent laboratory owners and operators. Their market for laboratory services outside the hospital is essentially targeted to physicians. They, not patients, order laboratory studies, so independent laboratories obviously depend on doctors for their business. Independent labs compete for this business on price, quality, timeliness of results, testing capability, and availability of courier pickup of specimens. While concerned that they might not make any money under a national fee schedule, they support the concept of uniform reimbursement for outpatient tests.

This is understandable because independent laboratories argue that hospitals and physicians have a competitive advantage in that they operate captive labs, dictating both the supply and demand for services. The independents are also the most highly regulated component of the laboratory market, and equal reimbursement should mean equal regulations. Congress may give these labs a sympathetic ear because of growing concern over varying standards in different clinical lab settings. One of the points the HCFA task force made was that testing differences in one setting versus another should be neutralized. Uniformity, HCFA felt, would reintroduce the physicians' offices and hospital laboratories to the competitive pressures that the independents feel.[8] Congressional committee staffs are now broaching the idea of a legislative proposal. With HCFA's encouragement, we may see legislation to require uniform Medicare standards applied across the board. Movement in this direction, however, would represent a marked departure from current Congressional support of a favored exempt status for physicians' office testing.

A variety of economic factors will continue to favor the growth in office testing. Reimbursement pressures on hospitals still make it advantageous for them to allow preadmission tests done in the doctor's office to be entered on the patient's hospital chart. Office-based physicians can potentially boost net income through operating efficiencies and better utilization of their own and office staff time, even with restrictive fee schedules. In addition, office lab testing can increase patient satisfaction by providing timely testing during single-visit consultations for most common medical problems. Since physicians' income is, to a great extent, a function of the number of patients they see, this competitive edge could be the overriding incentive to bring testing into the office.

PREDICTIONS

Federal regulatory agencies seem reluctant to license doctors' offices laboratories, seeing it as politically hazardous. But it is quite evident that the reimbursement shakedown for clinical laboratory services is far from over. As the volume and cost of laboratory testing increase, we can expect more government scrutiny and experimentation. Controls on doctors' office testing will likely come from private insurers in the form of restricted reimbursement to unregulated labs and from hospitals in restricted use of data from doctors' offices.

We also expect to see pathologists, technologists, chemists, and microbiologists entering into voluntary consultative relationships with doctors' office laboratories. Through educational and consulting services, they will help these facilities achieve a higher standard of practice.

REFERENCES

1. Halper RH, Foster HS: Regulation of physician office laboratories, Section 1.4, *Laboratory Regulation Manual Volume I*. Aspen Systems, Rockville, Md, 1976.

2. Halper RH, Foster HS: State laboratory programs, Section 5.1, *Laboratory Regulation Manual Volume II*. Aspen Systems, Rockville, Md, 1976.

3. Legislative Counsel's Digest, Chapter 960, Senate Bill No. 516, Section 4, Section 14105.3 of the Welfare and Institutions Code.

4. Belsey RE, Baer DM: Regulation of the SPOT Lab. *Clin Chem News* 1985;11(June suppl):20.

5. Crawley R, Belsey RE, Brock D, et al: Regulation of Physicians' Office Labs: The Idaho Experience. Submitted to *JAMA*.

6. Health Care Financing Administration: Laboratory Task Force Report, Memorandum to Carolyne Davis, Ph.D., Administrator, Feb 15, 1984, p 2.

7. American Academy of Family Physicians: Organization and Management of Family Practice: An Advisory Manual for the Family Physician in Private Practice, 1982.

8. Health Care Financing Administration: Laboratory Task Force Report, Memorandum to Carolyne Davis, Ph.D., Administrator, Feb 15, 1984, p 7.

9. Bartola J: Physician office lab reimbursement: Shifting strategies at the state level. Proceedings of the Second Annual Institute on Clinical Lab Reimbursement and Policy conducted by Washington G-2 Reports, Arlington, Va, Sept 7-8, 1984.

7

Malpractice and liability

When physicians expand their services into laboratory testing, their liability risk tends to grow apace, and they must ask themselves how they should manage this additional exposure. We will offer some suggestions in this chapter on managing the potential liability and implementing procedures and protocols to minimize the greater risk.

STANDARD OF CARE

Fundamentally, a malpractice case brought against a physician or medical provider is based on negligence, which is generally defined as conduct deviating from an expected standard of care. In addition, the following conditions must be met in order to prove negligence:

- the duty to perform certain services with accuracy,
- a breach of that duty,
- damage to the patient,
- a causal connection between the breach and the damage.

Traditionally, the question of a physician's negligence was evaluated by looking at the level of practice among peers in the community (known as the locality rule), but this narrow interpretation has recently been broadened. In 1979, a court determined that the medical personnel involved in the testing process, including the technicians performing the test and the physician interpreting it, were subject to a national standard since the tests were processed according to nationally standardized procedure protocols.[1] State-of-the-art methodology is thus becoming the yardstick by which the health-care professional's actions (including laboratory practice) will be judged. If the practitioner is a certified professional or uses certified technology—regardless of where this may be—then the standard of care will be established by national criteria and state-of-the-art technology. This legal evolution imposes a significant burden on practitioners to achieve a high level of performance.

A recent review of cases relating to laboratories' liability for test results confirmed the trend away from the locality rule and toward state-of-the-art standards for judging liability. Many of the cases concerned testing procedures for diabetes; today's more precise methods of glucose monitoring were clearly the state-of-the-art standards of care and were, in fact, already being applied.[2] As testing moves from the hospital to the office laboratory, the same performance criteria will follow.

POTENTIAL PLAINTIFFS

Another development that expands the scope of liability for laboratory professionals concerns who may find them negligent. Traditionally, the medical practitioner was responsible only to the patient, and not to any third party. A recent case involving negligence in testing for Tay-Sachs disease, however, held that physicians can be responsible to third parties, in this case to an unborn child. The child, who was unborn when the testing was done, was allowed to sue and recovered a substantial damage award as an intended beneficiary of the testing.[3] The important point here is that traditional limitations of responsibility solely to the patient may not apply. There is an inexorable movement of negligence law toward reasonable foreseeability in defining who is owed a duty of care. Not only is the patient the beneficiary of a medical provider's duty, but also anyone who may be reasonably foreseen to be affected by those actions.

BREACH OF DUTY

For negligence to exist, there must be a demonstrated breach of duty, and the law says the practitioner must fulfill this duty by reasonable efforts. An absolute standard does not apply. Instead, it becomes a question of determining what a reasonably prudent person of similar training and background and using similar technology would do in a situation. In the practice of laboratory testing, what procedures would a reasonably prudent technician follow? What calibration would be expected? What records should the technician complete and save? What information should be given to the patient?

DAMAGE

This is the third element in determining negligence—and damage means more than just obvious personal injury. There are, for example, slander cases because false gonorrhea reports damaged reputations. Other cases have cited serious emotional and psychological damage from erroneous test results. The ramifications of an erroneous test result can go beyond direct injury to the individual tested and beyond direct use of the result in patient management decisions. The potential for emotional and psychological injury, in particular, is very volatile.

An important issue concerning damage relates to the handling of mistakes. Since everyone makes mistakes at one time or another, the question of damages in a lawsuit can ultimately come down to how one handles the mistake. When negligence and damage have been established, an award can be markedly increased if the practitioners have concealed or changed records or ignored the problem and let it escalate. All too often a relatively nominal medical malpractice suit results in a larger award, which may include punitive damages, because of an apparent effort to ignore or hide an acknowledged mistake.

Medical records, another important issue here, help evaluate the range of damage that can result from a mistake. Complete records kept in a professional and organized manner may in fact show that the problem is probably nothing more than a mistake. They can show that there was no pattern of neglect or disregard for the patient's well-being. Good record keeping does not eliminate potential liability, but it can minimize the risk of larger or punitive damages being awarded.

CAUSATION

There are relatively few reported cases of laboratory liability. The reason is that the practicing clinicians are basically responsible for interpreting laboratory results. They receive the results and translate them into patient management decisions, presumably knowing the limitations of the testing process and of applying test results to patient care. Clinicians are interveners, that is, they cut off the laboratory's liability. The few cases reported usually include the clinician as a codefendant with the laboratorian.

In one case that resulted in a substantial judgment because of erroneous laboratory reports, the attending physician was held responsible for relying upon the quality of the results.[4] The more closely associated the physician is with those who perform the test, the more liable that physician will probably be for any mistakes.

If hospital or independent laboratory testing is replaced by testing done in the office laboratory, the physician's liability exposure will increase significantly. This change eliminates the laboratory's shield and puts the physician in the role of the professional who is both responsible and liable for the validity of the test result.

And the physician with an office laboratory should be aware of the legal theory called vicarious liability. This theory holds that employers are responsible for the negligent acts of their employees, whether or not they are present and whether or not they know what is going on, as long as the employee is working within the scope of the employment.[5] This requires the physician to have an organized system for training personnel, reporting test results, keeping records, and maintaining a quality-control system to monitor test results. The physician must also make sure that reported results have been processed appropriately and must monitor quality and maintain quality-assurance records in an ongoing fashion. The physician accepts professional responsibility when laboratory test processing is brought into his or her office.

Another area that involves potential liability exposure relates to integrating test results into the broader picture of diagnosis and management. The laboratory is one element of the traditional diagnostic troika: history, physical examination, and laboratory test results. Each contributes significantly but variably to the process. A number of recent cases have commented on today's tendency to rely too much on scientific testing. Several law review articles highlight the fact that as tests become more scientific, many medical practitioners rely totally and exclusively on a test result and fail to correlate such results with clinical observations or the history. It is important to remember that laboratory testing is only one part of the diagnostic and management equation and that total reliance on its absolute scientific accuracy is not prudent.

MANAGING LIABILITY RISK: PROCESS CONTROL

Liability in laboratory testing may fall on three persons:
- the one doing the test,
- the one conveying the test results, and
- the one interpreting the result and applying it to a patient-care decision.

Most readers are probably familiar with the elaborate preflight checkout that pilots perform before taking off. They want to make sure that everything is working right before departure—not while they're in the air!

The laboratory can also take some simple prophylactic measures to minimize error. First, it must have written, well-organized procedures for maintaining and calibrating equipment, for periodically verifying equipment accuracy, and for checking the proficiency of employees doing the tests. These procedures should be designed to provide early warning of problems before patient care is compromised.

Inasmuch as most laboratory mistakes are not immediately apparent, it is important to maintain records documenting the performance of quality-assurance procedures. This will provide supportive evidence if anyone makes allegations of an erroneous laboratory result. Physicians' office laboratories without such procedures and records, which we discuss in detail in Section III, enhance their liability risk.

A recent case involving an award of more than $900,000 against the clinician, hospital, and laboratory highlighted this particular problem. A jury found that an erroneous bilirubin result caused brain damage in an infant.[4] The reagent used to process the test was outdated and consequently produced a result lower than the actual value. Damaging evidence showed that there had been no regular, effective procedure to check reagent expiration dates.

MANAGING LIABILITY RISK: TEST REPORTING

A major issue in evaluating an alleged laboratory error involves confirmation that a certain specimen from a certain patient gave the questionable result. A common problem in large institutions is maintaining positive specimen identification throughout the collection, transportation, processing, and reporting cycle. Mislabeling a blood sample in one recent case led to an erroneous test report; the patient relied on it to make a decision regarding follow-up care and said it would have been different if the right result had been known.[6] Most laboratories mark the specimen with a unique number as well as with the patient's name and identification to make sure that the results are entered in the right record.

Although the office laboratory scale is smaller, patient identification still carries risk. For example, a physician may see a parent and a child, often with the same first and last name, on the same day and order laboratory tests. Positive identification for each specimen is essential, as is a system for recording the identification throughout the testing and reporting process to make sure that results are kept straight. It is useful to keep a master test log to record all requests (including a control number for identifying each specimen) and all results.

This approach, combined with instrument logs, makes it possible to trace a result reported at a particular time, step by step, back to the specimen collection, and to verify that the method or procedure was functional. These records facilitate evaluation of problems if results are reported for the wrong patient, and they let the clinician take early corrective action. In addition to minimizing their occurrence, the early reaction to and resolution of potential problems substantiate the office laboratory's professionalism.

MANAGING LIABILITY RISK: INTERPRETATION

This concerns the completeness of the patient's test report. Most medical negligence cases include an opening statement claiming that the doctor wouldn't talk to the patient, explain things, or answer questions. The lack of communication frequently stimulates a problem that need not exist. If a test result is reported to a patient, the doctor must make the patient understand that the results may have limitations and that alternative tests may be necessary to verify the result. This is especially true if the result is used as the basis for a major change in diagnosis or management.

In one case,[2] a urine result in the patient's chart showed a positive test for glucose. The doctor told the patient about the finding but did not advise her that a blood test was necessary to make the definitive diagnosis of diabetes. He was found negligent because he did not explain the limitations of the test and did not explain or do the appropriate follow-up test.

A similar liability risk exists for the physician in applying the test result to patient diagnosis or management. Many people believe that physicians cure disease and that if they visit a doctor they should be better afterward. They don't understand that bad results can occur through no one's negligence. This is one reason for explaining why the test is being done and describing its limitations.

The physician is also obliged to explain in a way that makes the patient understand. Such communication is critical to let the patient exercise whatever judgment is necessary on his or her own behalf—the legal requirement is informed consent, not merely consent. Communication also serves to build the kind of trusting relationship that most professionals want to have with the people they serve. Without such communication, the liability risk increases significantly.

REDUCING LIABILITY: RECORDS

Now that we have reviewed some issues of potential liability for the physician's office laboratory, we will turn to some concrete approaches toward minimizing the risk.

The vast majority of medical negligence cases are tried on records—or the lack of them. The operating assumption is that if it isn't written down, it wasn't done. Based on the age of documentation in which we live, that is a pretty reasonable assumption. It isn't enough to claim that "we always do it that way, so I'm sure that's what we did," when no specific record was made. Laboratory records contain the history of its performance and quality just as a patient's chart is the legal record of his or her treatment. Both chart and records must be complete.

From the legal perspective, records serve four purposes. First, they are a way to document what happened without reliance on memory—a memory confounded by trying to recall specific events about one incident out of hundreds and details of one set of circumstances out of thousands. Second, records serve as a point of reference to refresh the physician's memory and allow development of the facts necessary to explain a particular decision in patient care. Third, records help establish credibility in the eyes of anyone evaluating circumstances after the fact. It may be true that "it's always done that way," but a written record brings credibility. A well-written record is evidence that the physician's recall is correct, and at the same time, it reflects favorably on his or her professional demeanor. There is nothing more unprofessional looking than a disorganized, incomplete medical record. Finally, records minimize the cost of a physician's mistakes. As a practical matter, they can let a jury see that a physician may have made a mistake but was not irresponsible, a finding that can save dollars and embarrassment.

What is the minimal documentation needed for office laboratory testing? First, it is essential to develop a way to document the proper functioning of the laboratory systems and equipment. This includes a patient log with the patient's name and identification, tests ordered, and results reported (in addition to the lab report in the patient's medical record). Second, there should be an equipment maintenance, calibration, and troubleshooting log, which includes a record of recalibration and problems with each instrument, providing a complete profile of machine or system performance. Third is the procedure manual, which details the specific techniques for performing a test. Finally, the testing log lists all tests performed on a particular piece of equipment. It includes the values of control sera used to identify early signs of a system malfunction and written evidence of any action taken to evaluate or correct the problem.

Another document important in the office laboratory is a procedure checklist. Someone who does a test usually does it the same way every time. But as time passes, the person may modify the procedure slightly and produce a result that is close to, but not identical with, the original procedure. The familiar procedure then starts to deviate more and more from the standard, and the end result is a change in overall accuracy.

A variation on this theme is that one person will perform the test following a procedure learned in one setting, and another will do it, as learned, somewhat differently. This is particularly dangerous because a test's operating characteristics may vary greatly between the two and give markedly different results with the same specimen. It is thus essential to have a checklist at the work station with the approved procedure for each test done in the laboratory. A complete procedure check should also be done periodically, depending on testing volume and the nature of the systems being used, but at least once a year.

These records are potentially a double-edged sword because an attorney could use the procedure checklist, for example, to interrogate laboratory personnel. If the documentation is incomplete or a step is missing, it could be a serious problem. On the other hand, the only way to ensure the continuity and uniformity of laboratory practice is to maintain these records and keep them up to date. The benefits far outweigh the risks. It is also important for the responsible physician to review these records, including a periodic review and update of the procedure manual and of personnel performance. Records of such reviews should be kept to document the laboratory's efforts at maintaining a uniform, reliable level of proficiency. This kind of information goes a long way toward reducing and managing liability potential.

Such records must be kept even after the testing systems are no longer used. With the rapid evolution of technology, the actual life of any piece of equipment depends on its usability, and the potential liability problem may not even surface until after a machine has been discarded. Records should be kept for a reasonable period of time (depending on the state's laws) to provide some history of the machine's function even though the instrument itself is no longer available.

REDUCING LIABILITY: IN-SERVICE EDUCATION

Each laboratory must have a program of regular in-service education. The physician or the office manager should require continuing education as a condition of employment of anyone performing tests. This should be encouraged by such incentives as allowing employees paid time and support to attend classes or providing learning opportunities in the office during regular work hours. This will let them keep up with recent developments and refresh established knowledge and skills.

It is also useful to keep personnel records that document the employee's proficiency in performing tests and detailed evidence of ongoing training to maintain those skills, including the date, site, sponsoring organization, and subject matter of each class or workshop. As we noted in the discussion on records, in-service or continuing education gives further support to the laboratory's professionalism and its claims that appropriate techniques were used to perform tests. Continuing education entails a relatively small investment of time and money, but it has a big impact on how well the laboratory performs.

MANAGING LIABILITY EXPOSURE: DON'TS

Among the most important elements in minimizing liability is the attitude and philosophy that the physician's office has about testing. Here are a few comments that may help establish an appropriate climate.

Don't be defensive. We all know that people have the tendency to justify decisions by subsequent acts and hindsight thinking. It is far more important to develop good quality-control guidelines that have the support of the laboratory staff than to justify the procedures as they exist. It is also important to remain relatively open and objective about modifying the quality-control guidelines if necessary. If a test system is properly used and calibrated and if the physician can explain how it works so that it is understood, that is enough. Being professional is more important than being defensive. Defensive medicine leads to mistakes that cause more serious problems.

Don't cover up. If there's a problem, deal with it and solve it. It is shortsighted to think that writing down the problem is tantamount to admitting fault and liability. A mistake is a mistake, and a cover-up attempt can only magnify the problem. The really serious problems begin if a cover-up becomes apparent. It escalates the cost both in terms of dollars and the physician's personal reputation.

Don't ignore problems. They don't go away—they just get much more serious. So if a staff member has trouble doing a certain test or if there's a stability problem with calibrating an instrument, deal with it promptly.

Don't be secretive. Tell the patient the purpose of the test, any limitations of the result, and any recommendations concerning verification or follow-up. This applies across the board, from the most common to the most exotic tests. Most people know, for example, what a biopsy is supposed to show, but very few understand its limitations.

The physician must communicate on two levels: 1) with the employee on collecting the specimen, performing the test, and reporting the results; and 2) with the patient on the need, rationale, limitations, results, and interpretation of the test. Both are essential in managing potential liability.

CONCLUSION

New technology creates new responsibilities and new liability risks for medical negligence. Mistakes are bound to occur, but an organized system along the lines suggested in this chapter is a workable way to minimize the number of mistakes and the consequences of any that do occur. The benefit—both to the physician and to the patient—far outweighs the risk of using the new technology and procedures.

REFERENCES

1. *Morrison v MacNamara*, 407 A2d 555 (DC App 1979). This case involved a urethral smear test by a nationally certified clinical medical laboratory. The court held that a national standard was the measure of the standard of care "at least as to board-certified physicians, hospitals, medical laboratories, and other health care providers." Compare *Ries v Reinard*, 114 P2d 386 (Cal App 1941).

2. In *Dowell v Mossberg*, 355 P2d 624 (Ore 1961), a chiropractic physician was affirmed negligent for not following up a suspicious urine test for glucose with a blood glucose test. The court ruled that a person who held himself out as competent to diagnose diabetes was required to use widely recognized and accepted diagnostic testing.

3. *Curlender v Bio-Science Laboratories*, 165 Cal Rpts 477 (Cal App 1980). Here the court permitted a "wrongful life" action for a defective child to proceed because of "incorrect and inaccurate" information given the parents concerning their status as genetic carriers of Tay-Sachs disease.

4. In *Schnibly v Baker*, 217 NW2 708 (Iowa 1974), the court affirmed a verdict of $912,124 against the pediatricians, the hospital, and the laboratory pathologists for improper bilirubin tests because of the use of outdated reagents.

5. In *Lazevnick* v *General Hospital of Monroe County*, 499 F. Supp. 146 (CA Pa 1980), the court held that the pathologist in charge of the hospital's laboratory department could be held responsible for a lab technician's error even though the pathologist was not a hospital employee.

6. In *Naccash v Burger*, 290 SE 2d 825 (Va 1982), parents of a child born with Tay-Sachs disease were allowed to recover for "wrongful birth" because of mislabeling of blood sample that made the parents decide not to abort the fetus.

8

Cost accounting

In this chapter we want to acquaint the physician interested in doing office laboratory testing with the actual costs of doing so. This information is essential in deciding whether to do office testing or send it out to a reference laboratory.

If the revenue generated from doing the tests is significantly greater than the cost of producing the results, there may be financial as well as clinical incentives for developing an office laboratory. On the other hand, if the projected revenue is significantly less than the cost, there will be a distinct financial disincentive for the office laboratory. And in some circumstances, good clinical reasons, such as the timely availability of results in managing a difficult case, might justify doing them in the office even if the revenue does not equal the cost. Many factors must go into the decision; cost is but one of them.

MAJOR CATEGORIES OF EXPENSE

We will analyze each of the six major sources of expenses for laboratory testing so as to derive the annualized costs of performing tests based upon the volume of testing generated. They follow here.

Supplies consist of materials used to collect specimens—blood, urine, and spinal fluid—plus reagents, calibrators, and disposables (such as test tubes and pipettes) used for test processing. Supply costs are directly related to the volume of specimens obtained and tests performed.

Labor costs. Chemists, medical technologists, nurses, receptionists, and even physicians can perform laboratory tests. If the person performs other duties, the labor costs of lab testing should be prorated accordingly. Labor costs are incremental and rise in stair-step fashion. They are not linearly related to but are a function of test volume.

Depreciation, the mechanism used to spread capital expenditure over the useful life of the equipment, can be done several ways. But either straight-line or declining depreciation schedules have been most commonly used for laboratory equipment. With a straight-line schedule, a constant fraction of the total cost is allocated to each year of the equipment's expected life; for example, it's 20% a year for an instrument with an expected five-year life.

The simplest declining depreciation schedule involves allocating a fixed fraction of the capital expense balance, after deducting depreciation expense from previous years, so that the total remaining balance is depreciated during the last year of expected equipment life. Declining depreciation for an instrument with an expected five-year useful life might be 33% of the outstanding capital balance each year with the remainder depreciated during the fifth year. Selecting a depreciation schedule obviously has significant implications with regard to offsetting taxable income. The doctor may wish to consult with a banker, a financial adviser, or tax consultant for expert advice.

Interest The cost of borrowing capital must also be included in the operating costs of an instrument or system. What is not widely appreciated is that a cash purchase, particularly of expensive equipment, means losing investment capital. This should therefore be included in any analysis as an expense that can be allocated to operating the test system.

Maintenance is the cost of preventive maintenance and repair services, including the cost of replacement parts. This will vary, depending upon the type of system as well as the specific coverage required (eight hours a day, six days a week, say, compared with 24 hours a day, 365 days a year). Annual maintenance cost is usually figured at 10% of the initial capital investment.

Quality control (QC) expenses include the cost of the control material and the additional reagent and labor costs to perform these tests, plus the estimated cost of any repeat testing necessitated by "out-of-control" results. Estimated QC expenditures will depend upon the number of different assays being performed and the cost of their reagents. It may also vary with the particular instrument being used; some are intrinsically more stable or less subject to operator or system errors. QC cost is more fixed than variable; it is not related to the number of daily tests, but is rather a function of the type of assays performed.

ANALYZING COSTS: SOME EXAMPLES

The estimated cost of doing 30, 60, 90, 120, 150, or 180 tests a day is shown in Table 8-1. The clinician who knows the potential utilization of office testing can use this table as a guideline for estimating the cost of maintaining that laboratory. We will discuss two of these cases, 30 and 120 tests daily, in some detail to familiarize the reader with the estimation process. Financial analysis for evaluating a specific doctor's office lab will depend on developing applicable information for that setting.

We will assume that the tests are performed for 10 different patients and that each request averages three tests ordered. For each venipuncture, we will assume that blood drawing supplies cost $1.25, or $12.50 for the 10 patients. We estimate that reagents and disposables cost $2 per test or $60 per day. Arbitrarily assuming that the venipunctures and test processing will require 4.8 hours of employee time (0.6 of a full day's work) at an estimated salary and fringe benefit cost of $100, the labor would cost $60 daily. Thus the direct cost of supplies and labor to produce the 30 results per day would be $132.50, about $4.46 for each test result reported. Assuming 250 work days per year, the annualized direct cost of producing these tests is $33,125.

Assuming a capital investment of $6,000 for this small laboratory, the depreciation and interest expenses amount to $2,000 a year, and maintenance costs are estimated at $600 annually. The QC cost, including control material and reagents can be estimated at $8,000 per year. Total expenses to process this test volume are estimated to be $43,725 per year, or $5.83 for each result reported.

As testing volume increases, the cost of producing each result will go down because of economies of scale and spreading fixed costs over the greater number of tests. Using the same approach as before with 120 tests per day, the annualized costs for

TABLE 8-1

Annualized cost analysis as a function of test volume

	Number of physicians					
	1	2	3	4	5	6
Tests per day	30	60	90	120	150	180
Patients per day	10	20	30	40	50	60
Costs per day						
Supplies						
Specimen collection ($1.25 per patient)	$ 12.50	25.00	37.50	50.00	62.50	75.00
Reagents and disposables ($2 per test)	$ 60.00	120.00	180.00	240.00	300.00	360.00
Labor 1 FTE = $100 per day	.6 FTE $ 60.00	1 FTE 100.00	1.4 FTE 140.00	1.7 FTE 170.00	1.85 FTE 185.00	2 FTE 200.00
Supplies and labor	$132.50	245.00	357.50	460.00	547.50	635.00
Costs per year						
Supplies and labor	$33,125	61,250	89,375	115,000	136,875	158,750
Depreciation (B)*	$ 2,000	3,000	4,000	5,000	6,000	6,666
Maintenance (C)	$ 600	900	1,200	1,500	1,800	2,000
Quality control (D)	$ 8,000	10,000	12,000	14,000	16,000	16,000
Total (A + B + C + D)	**$43,725**	**75,150**	**106,575**	**135,500**	**160,675**	**183,416**

*This assumes a capital outlay for instrument systems of $6,000, $9,000, $12,000, $15,000, $18,000, or $20,000, respectively, for the six cases in the table.

supplies and labor would be $115,000 and for the QC program, maintenance, interest, and depreciation expenses would be about $20,500. The total annualized cost is estimated at $135,500 ($4.52 for each reported result).

With increased volume, two opportunities might exist. First, the physician might be able to negotiate a quantity discount on the cost of supplies, significantly reducing the reagent cost per test. Second, an alternative, more economical, approach to test processing might become feasible. The annualized $4.52 per reported result might well be an overestimate that could be cut with careful management.

ANALYZING REVENUE: SOME EXAMPLES

Reimbursement formulas for ambulatory-care testing have recently been subject to significant changes and will probably remain volatile for some time (Chapter 6). It is also important to remember that reimbursement rates for office laboratory testing vary considerably, depending on the geographic area and the nature of the patient's insurance coverage. For these examples, we will consider four different reimbursement schedules—$4, $6, $8, and $10 per result—and make the following assumptions: The reimbursement for specimen collection and handling is $3 per specimen, three tests per specimen are ordered, and the laboratory is open 250 days a year. Table 8-2 shows the estimated reimbursement for the test volumes used in the earlier examples with discussion in the following paragraphs.

Total reimbursement for a laboratory producing 30 results a day would be $37,500 ($4 per test), $52,500 ($6 per test), $67,500 ($8 per test), and $82,500 ($10 per test). With the estimated cost of producing these test results being $43,725, all but the lowest schedule would be quite profitable. If the laboratory charges $8 per test (a reasonable estimate for many practices) and $3 per specimen for collecting and handling, net revenue would be about $25,000 a year.

For a laboratory processing 120 tests a day, the total revenues would project from $150,000 to $330,000 annually, depending upon the reimbursement level. Again assuming reimbursement of $8 per test and $3 for specimen collection and handling, the net revenue would be about $135,000, or $35,000 per practitioner in a four-physician group.

Annualized revenue analysis as a function of test volume and reimbursement

Tests per day*	Per-test charge†			
	$4	$6	$8	$10
30	$ 37,500	$ 52,500	$ 67,500	$ 82,500
60	75,000	105,000	135,000	165,000
90	112,500	157,500	202,000	247,500
120	150,000	210,000	270,000	330,000
150	187,500	262,500	337,500	412,500
180	225,000	315,000	405,000	492,500

*Assume three tests per specimen and 250 working days per year
† Plus $3 per test for specimen collection

CONCLUSION

Cost accounting is critically important in deciding whether or not to do testing in an office laboratory. A number of programs are available for the IBM-PC, Apple II series, and other personal computers that will let physicians estimate practice expenses and determine the break-even point for various procedures with different reimbursement schedules. Obviously, financial considerations are but one factor in making such a decision, but we hope the information in this chapter has helped you understand them.

GENERAL REFERENCE

1. Schroeder SA, Showstack JA: Financial incentives to perform medical procedures and laboratory tests: Illustrative models of office practice. *Med Care* 1978;16:289-298.

The analytical practice of office testing

9

Setting up the laboratory

The principles of planning a laboratory are essentially the same regardless of setting. Such details as location, size, essential utilities, communications, design of working and storage areas, and the need for eventual expansion must be considered at the outset because renovation and the attendant disruption of patient care are quite difficult. The key decisions are related to allowing enough space, providing a convenient layout, and most important, providing a setting conducive to quality testing. Employees involved in the testing cycle must have room to collect specimens, process them, and report test results.

LOCATION

The laboratory and a conveniently located lavatory should be close to the waiting room. In a large group practice or emergency clinic, it may be useful to cluster the laboratory, x-ray facilities, and pharmacy.

SIZE

There are few good guidelines to help plan laboratory size, but certain key functions must be provided for. Space for drawing blood specimens is essential, and there must be counters to accommodate equipment, shelves to store specimens, and files for record keeping. Different settings obviously require vastly different amounts of space.

Also important is the most efficient use of space; many planners consider it to be rooms or modules 10 by 20 feet, a shape that provides up to 45 linear feet of counter space. In a typical arrangement, counters are two and a half feet deep with aisles five feet wide. This gives one or more employees room to move without wasting floor space. Free-standing equipment such as refrigerators and blood-drawing chairs can replace counter area. If more space is required, a second module of the same dimensions can be added. In our experience, three such modules are about right for a group practice clinic with 24 to 36 physicians.

To determine the appropriate amount of space for your setting, it will help to make a list of all the equipment your lab will need. List the size of each instrument and necessary working space around it. Don't forget refrigerators, file cabinets, clerical areas, and blood-drawing stations, with their associated supplies and work areas. Sinks and counters for washing and draining glassware should also be provided.

Most planners we've talked to agree on several basic principles of forecasting laboratory space requirements:

- Every laboratory will eventually be too small;
- There are no good guidelines for making space forecasts;
- Any forecast will probably be inaccurate.

In view of this, it is probably wise to allow for more space than your forecast predicts. This will let you add equipment—or provide for what you forgot in your projections. It is also wise to plan for expansion from the beginning. Perhaps a good-sized storage closet could be included, for example. Expansion should also be considered in plumbing and electrical plans.

TOILETS

A lavatory should be convenient to the lab, perhaps in the same corridor. A pass-through window is one way to let patients place a urine specimen directly in the lab without having to walk through a waiting area with it. Depending on the practice, you may want to have toilet facilities for the handicapped and allow for wheelchairs in the lavatory. All doors should be wide enough to accommodate wheelchairs.

CABINETS

Certain tests—on chemistry analyzers or blood cell counters, for example—are traditionally performed standing up, while others—with microscopes—are easier to do sitting down. For this reason, two cabinet heights (29 to 30 inches for sitting and 36 to 37 inches for standing) should be provided, with appropriate knee space. We have found that a putty- or clay-colored countertop with a high-pressure, laminated plastic matte finish is both attractive and utilitarian. For upper and lower cabinets and chairs, we like attractive colors that fit the office decorating scheme. Upper cabinets, preferably with solid doors and adjustable shelves, provide important storage space. They may be 12 to 18 inches deep; lower cabinets are usually 24 to 30 inches deep.

Although adjustable shelves are convenient for upper cabinets, most of the lower ones should have drawers ranging from three to nine or 10 inches deep. Shelves are wasteful even for large objects, since only the front is easily accessible. Drawers, on the other hand, provide complete access. In designing a drawer system, you may want to arrange the tracks so that the drawers can be interchanged between cabinets. Some cabinet designs put drawers of utilitarian design behind a more decorative door. If you're considering them, pay special attention to the hinge design. You should not have to open the door a full 180 degrees in order to pull out the drawer.

Chairs and stools for the technologists should be comfortable and provide good back support. Each employee should have a chair.

Several manufacturers make blood-drawing chairs that allow good support for the arm and security against falling if the patient should feel faint. Remember, too, that you may have to draw specimens from patients in wheelchairs, and plan the blood-drawing area accordingly.

UTILITIES

The most important utility is electrical power, which almost all laboratory instruments require. A common problem is not having enough outlets; one good way to provide them is with plug-mold strips with outlets every six inches. They should be mounted several inches above the counter along each wall, but not on the counter itself where spills can occur. On counters with no walls behind them, use double-sided, four-plex receptacles at six-foot intervals. Twenty-ampere circuits are necessary for such heavy-drain equipment as refrigerators and centrifuges, and sensitive electronic instruments like blood cell counters should also have separate circuits.

One of the deficiencies that accrediting agencies find most frequently in doctors' office laboratories is inadequate light. It is often so poor that evaluating color changes on dipsticks becomes impossible. Ceiling fixtures with natural color balance fluorescent tubes are desirable, at an intensity of about 75 foot candles of light at the countertop. Nor should the light be too bright or glaring. Continuous, single-fluorescent strips under the upper cabinets with a diffusing device or an indirect lighting baffle can provide shadow-free illumination at the counters.

As for plumbing, a small laboratory should have a sink for dishwashing and specimen disposal. It should be near the blood-drawing area so that phlebotomists can easily wash their hands. If the laboratory has more than one module, there should be a sink for each one—at the bottom of the U-shaped counter area is most convenient. Most building codes require vacuum breakers on laboratory faucets. Accrediting agencies also require eye-wash stations and a drench shower, in case of fire or chemical spill. A spray attachment at the sink is the easiest way to handle this.

Adequate air conditioning and ventilation are too often overlooked in doctors' office labs, but they are essential for removing toxic fumes, unpleasant odors, and the heat that laboratory instruments generate. Refrigerators, centrifuges, electronic instruments, and incubators produce a lot of heat. The laboratory requires much more ventilation than waiting or examining rooms and should have its own thermostatic control. Gas, air, or vacuum lines are seldom required in doctors' office laboratories. If tuberculosis or fungal tests are performed, a biological safety hood must be used when doing them; an electric incinerator can be used to sterilize the bacteriology plating loop or needle.

AMENITIES

It is important to make a small laboratory a pleasant place to spend one's working hours. Some communication with the outside world—a window or skylight— helps, especially if the room is small. Color in the walls, furnishings, cabinetry, and floor is also a plus. Employees will need coat racks and lockers for personal belongings, and they will also appreciate having a small refrigerator for their lunches, since accrediting agencies prohibit food in refrigerators that store specimens or reagents. If space permits, a bulletin board and wall clock are also nice touches.

ARCHITECTURAL ASPECTS OF SAFETY

Unless open flames are used—and electric incinerators and hot plates are preferable—fire hazard is probably quite low. High-pressure plastic laminate on countertops and cabinets is fire resistant and more durable than wood. Wooden floors are also undesirable. They are more flammable, cleaning is more difficult, and they are less durable and subject to staining. Composition flooring in sheets is easiest to clean, as well as less fatiguing to stand on. Any curtains or drapes should be fire resistant.

Safety rules require that flammable liquids in amounts greater than one pint must be kept in metal safety cabinets that are usually vented to the outside. Such liquids should be in metal containers and preferably in those of specific safety design. They should never be kept in an ordinary refrigerator; and even though evaporation may be somewhat greater, such flammable liquids as ether are more safely stored in a well-ventilated cabinet or countertop at room temperature.

A single entrance and exit to the laboratory is usually enough unless the area is very large or a number of people work in it. Fire exits from the laboratory and from the building should be clearly marked and well known to the employees. You may also want to refer to Chapter 11, which deals with safety.

ELECTRICAL SAFETY

All electrical circuits should be grounded according to electrical codes. Except for such equipment as lamps, all instruments should have three wire-grounded circuits. It is a good idea to check all outlets with an electrical ground tester to be sure that the wires have been installed properly. A high proportion of circuits, even those put in by qualified electricians, are improperly grounded or have the hot and neutral wires reversed. Circuits in areas close to sinks and where the operator may be exposed to an electrical appliance while being grounded should have ground fault interrupters. Frayed cords and other defective electrical appliances should be repaired promptly. Electrical circuits should not be overloaded by extension cords with many devices attached to them.

REFERENCES

1. Baer DM: Designing your laboratory, in Stefanini M: *Progress in Clinical Pathology, Vol VI*. New York, Grune & Stratton, 1975.

2. *CAP Manual for Laboratory Planning and Design,* College of American Pathologists, Skokie, Ill, 1977.

10

Personnel

$\mathbf{T}$he quality of a laboratory's work depends exclusively on its employees. Good and bad laboratories use the same equipment, the same reagents, and the same supplies. The difference between them lies in the people who care for the machines and perform the tests.

WHO IS DOING THE TESTS?

Today, individuals with widely different backgrounds and training are doing tests in physicians' office laboratories. They range from medical assistants with minimal on-the-job training to certified medical technologists who have studied the theory and practice of laboratory testing. Two studies of who does physicians' office testing[1,2] showed that 30% are technologists or technicians, 30% have been educated on the job, while 40% have no formal training in laboratory medicine. In order to assign duties and responsibilities appropriately, the physician should understand the differences in training and qualifications of office laboratory workers.

Medical technologist, MT(ASCP). This is someone who graduated from a baccalaureate-level medical technology program, including a full year of theoretical and practical training, and also passed a national certifying examination given by the Board of Registry of the American Society of Clinical Pathologists

(ASCP). These technologists should be able to perform laboratory tests requiring considerable skill and independent judgment; and after acquiring some experience they may become supervisors. Several other organizations also certify technologists.

Medical laboratory technician, MLT(ASCP). This is a graduate of a two-year associate degree program, of which a year is devoted to theory and practice. Certification requires passing a national examination, and these technicians can be expected to do many laboratory tests. Some regulatory agencies exclude them from doing tests that require independent judgment, such as microbiology tests and more advanced hematologic procedures requiring cell identification. An MLT is not expected to become a supervisor.

Certified laboratory assistant, CLA(ASCP). This is a graduate of a one-year program, usually given in a community college, that covers theory and practice of clinical laboratory procedures, and the designation is awarded after passing a national certification examination. Several certifying organizations give examinations at this level, designating those who pass as technicians. They are not expected to perform tests requiring exercise of independent judgment.

Medical office assistant. Some medical assistant programs that last anywhere from six months to a year may include laboratory training. One such program in a community college includes 80 hours of theoretical and practical instruction in drawing blood and preparing specimens to be sent to other laboratories, doing dipstick urinalyses, blood cell counting, plating bacteriology specimens, and performing Gram stains.

Nurse. Some nurses are proficient in venipuncture and skin puncture techniques, but few have been trained in the requirements and pitfalls of specimen collection. Formal training in doing basic laboratory tests is minimal in most nursing education programs.

Physician. Laboratory medicine education in medical school focuses on test interpretation, and only rarely does it include test analysis or quality control of the testing process.

SELECTING PERSONNEL TO DO OFFICE LAB TESTING

The choice of who should do the testing depends on its volume and complexity. Even the simplest procedure requires compulsive attention to detail and appreciation of the pitfalls it presents.

The technician must follow instructions faithfully and not experiment with shortcuts. Since many analyses require visual color comparisons, anyone who does them should be tested to make sure he or she is not color blind and can discern subtle color changes.

Some states have laboratory licensing laws that require specific training or certification for office lab personnel (Chapter 6, Regulation and reimbursement). If your hospital permits test results from an office laboratory to be entered in the patient's hospital chart, the office technician may be subject to training or certification requirements determined by the institution.

It may be difficult to assess an individual's ability to perform office lab testing, and you might want to ask your hospital's laboratory director to help you judge a job applicant's level of training, skill, and experience. Or you might ask a certified medical technologist who is already a member of your staff or temporarily hired for the purpose to observe the new employee, training him or her in basic testing techniques, the use and care of equipment, quality-assurance protocols, and the importance of careful and complete record-keeping.

OPPORTUNITIES FOR LABORATORY TRAINING

As we discuss in the chapter on liability, training is an essential part of any laboratory quality-assurance program. In-service education is important for people in any laboratory setting and regardless of previous laboratory training and experience. Keeping up is the name of the game.

What training opportunities are available for employees with no laboratory experience? One is a local hospital or independent laboratory whose personnel might give some training. Another is equipment and reagent manufacturers who frequently provide on-site training in using their products. One manufacturer of chemistry test systems, for instance, sends a qualified technologist to the doctor's office lab to install the equipment and train the staff in its operation, often for as long as half a day. If a change in staff requires additional training, it's done at no additional cost. Still another possibility is manufacturers who sponsor workshops that provide more formal educational programs. Finally, some professional societies and government agencies offer workshops or teleconferences that are appropriate for office laboratory workers. Among them are the ASCP, the Colorado Association for Continuing Laboratory Education, Centers for Disease Control, and state health departments.

As we also point out in the liability chapter, it is important to document the level of education, experience, special on-the-job instruction, and continuing education of the office laboratory staff. For those who lack specific laboratory training, it may also be appropriate to indicate which procedures each employee is qualified to perform. If someone has received training in operating an instrument, for example, say so in his or her personnel folder. Everyone who performs venipuncture should have to demonstrate proficiency in the technique, and the physician should authorize nonprofessional employees to perform such procedures with documentation in their personnel files.

WORKING ENVIRONMENT

Environment has a direct effect on the quality of work produced. In order to produce accurate test results, a person must be able to carry out a sequence of steps without interruption and devote full attention to the process. If the testing is a part-time task, that individual should be able to set aside a block of time that is free of distractions. A nurse or receptionist might not be appropriate, for example, particularly if he or she is frequently called away to perform other duties that are considered more important—such as those involving physician or patient interaction.

The physical environment also bears directly on the quality of testing. Adequate space, lighting, ventilation, and temperature control are necessary for the best performance. As we discuss in Chapter 9, lighting is particularly important in reading the subtle color changes in reagent dipstick chemistry systems (urine chemistry tests and capillary glucose testing).

REFERENCES

1. Brock DW, Crawley R, Anderson G, et al: An analysis of Idaho private physician office laboratory facilities and testing activities through on-site inspection. Centers for Disease Control, Contract 200-77-0716, 1977.

2. Gwyther RE, Kirkman-Liff BL: Laboratory testing in the offices of family physicians. *Am J Med Tech* 1982;48:697-702.

11

Safety

The development of clinical laboratories in physicians' offices brings new potential hazards to patients and office personnel alike. The physician responsible for operating the office laboratory must be aware of these hazards and try to minimize the risk. Among the risks are the testing systems themselves, which have potential chemical and electrical hazards, the greater numbers of patient specimens, and performing microbiological tests. The last two, of course, increase the risk of infection among the staff. In the hospital setting, these issues are the responsibility of the infection control officer and the hospital safety officer who are supported by interdepartmental multidiscipline committees.

A major focus of almost all laboratory accreditation programs is an evaluation of a lab's safety program, policies, and practice. The purposes of this chapter are to review potential hazards posed by the office laboratory and to help you reduce injury potential for office staff and patients. You may also want to refer to the safety section of the chapter dealing with office laboratory design (Chapter 9).

GENERAL SAFETY PRACTICES

Professional laboratorians almost universally accept some practices as essential for safe lab operation. First, lab-associated hazards should be confined to the laboratory area, and people who aren't aware of the risks should be kept out. Laboratorians uniformly agree that it is hazardous to drink (even water), eat, or smoke in the laboratory, so employees should have another convenient area for breaks and lunch. Food should never be stored in refrigerators used for patient specimens, laboratory reagents, or culture media.

It is generally appreciated that high places and transport can cause accidents. In the laboratory these risks translate into accidents from retrieving materials stored out of ordinary reach and from careless specimen handling or transport. The former can be avoided if materials, especially heavy ones, are stored within easy reach of someone standing at floor level. If this isn't always possible, a sturdy ladder or step ladder must be available. Employees should not lift or move heavy equipment alone, but should use a suitable dolly or hand truck. If they must lift a heavy object, they should use the proper stance—with the trunk erect and with the actual lifting done by straightening the legs. Finally, specimens should always be placed in a rack for transporting from one place to another, and it's safest to avoid carrying other objects at the same time.

CHEMICAL HAZARDS

The storage and use of chemical reagents may result in a variety of hazards—primarily an increased risk of being burned or affected by toxic fumes. Knowing the properties of the reagents and how to handle them will minimize the risk of accidents. First and foremost, mouth pipetting must never be used. Second, only a minimum amount of hazardous reagents should be stored in the office laboratory. Many of the new testing systems feature unit packaging, but if it's necessary to buy reagents in bulk, keep only limited quantities in the lab. If volatile materials are stored in the office, the quantity should be as small as possible, and storage facilities with a spark hazard (unmodified household refrigerators and freezers, for example) should be avoided. Containers for the storage of specimens, culture media, and reagents should be clearly labeled with the contents and any associated hazards.

Many newer chemistry testing systems feature unitized dry reagents, but some instruments being marketed to physicians' office laboratories are conventional wet chemistry systems in new packages. Caustic reagents are not hazardous so long as they are confined to the test tube, but they can easily cause burns if they are spilled or the test tubes break. Cleanup procedures, including the waste container of many chemistry analyzers, and treatment of anyone splashed with caustic materials, should be clearly detailed in the laboratory safety manual.

ELECTRICAL HAZARDS

Wherever there are electrical wires and connections there is the potential for shock and fire hazards. The external wiring of all instruments must be periodically inspected, and worn wires replaced. Electrical equipment and connections should not be handled with wet hands since some instruments are not adequately grounded or may have an internal current leak. Analytic instruments should be installed with three-prong (grounded) plugs, and if there is a shortage of outlets, it is much safer to install additional service than to use extension cords or multiple tap plugs in the duplex wall outlet.

As we noted, electrical equipment with spark hazards, especially switches and motors, should not be used where flammable vapors might be present. If volatile solvents are necessary, they should be kept at room temperature in a well-ventilated area, and the electrical equipment should be modified and checked to be sure it is explosion proof.

FIRE SAFETY

The laboratory should be organized for easy exit in case of fire. Fire extinguishers should be kept in or near the laboratory to handle small, contained fires, but with any larger fire, safe practice requires notifying the fire department immediately and evacuating the area. The guiding principle of fire safety should be to protect employees and patients from possible harm.

Despite the limited use of fire-fighting equipment in the laboratory, extinguishers should be well maintained and tested, and employees should know how to use them. A fire blanket should also be available. The lab staff should understand the hazards of using liquid extinguishers on instruments or when live electrical connections are exposed. There should be periodic drills to ensure that employees know how to respond to a fire and use the equipment properly. Although this seems disruptive to daily routine, it minimizes the hazard of serious injury. Local fire departments are usually glad to instruct people in the use of fire safety equipment.

TECHNIQUES FOR PREVENTING LABORATORY INFECTIONS

A major hazard in any health-care setting is infectious disease and exposure to infectious agents from patient specimens. An infection control program in the office setting should include appropriate immunization of the staff. Hepatitis B immunization is recommended for all laboratory personnel, and rubella immunization should be offered to female employees of child-bearing age and male employees with wives in this age group. If patients are known to be a contagious risk, their medical record jackets and laboratory request slips should be prominently marked to let the staff exercise appropriate caution (wearing gloves when handling serum specimens from hepatitis B patients, for example).

Another potential source of laboratory-acquired infection is the aerosolization of infectious material during sample preparation and test processing. Specimen containers should be checked for cracks before centrifugation and, when possible, stoppered during the process. Aerosols produced when excess blood is expelled from the needle tip can be minimized if the syringe is held vertically and the blood deposited directly into a cotton pledget. Plunging a flamed bacteriologic tip into a culture before it has cooled adequately is another source of potentially infectious aerosols that can be avoided with proper technique. Cleaning and maintenance procedures should include periodic decontamination of areas exposed to infectious materials. We'll discuss disposing of infectious waste in the next section.

Much of the responsibility for avoiding infection rests with the employee. The office should have an active safety program, as we'll discuss in a moment. As part of this program, employees working with potentially infectious material should be taught to keep their hands away from their face, eyes, nose, and mouth to prevent self-inoculation. They should also be taught that frequent hand washing during the day is an easy, efficient way to reduce the potential for carrying and being infected with a potential pathogen. Serum separated from blood should not be decanted but should be transferred by pipette, and never by mouth pipetting. And as we said, there must be no eating, drinking, or smoking in the laboratory.

LABORATORY WASTE DISPOSAL

A laboratory creates potentially hazardous waste. And although it is important to establish procedures for its proper disposal, prevention is a more effective approach to reducing the risk of injury. For example, disposing of intact and broken glass poses a significant hazard to the cleaning people and office staff. It is better to segregate glass from paper and other solid waste and put it in clearly marked containers for separate disposal. Another approach is to replace glass equipment and supplies with plastic whenever possible.

Another problem is the disposal of blood, urine, and stool specimens. The office staff is probably used to disposing of needles and syringes, but it has always sent the specimens to a reference laboratory for analysis and disposal. Liquid and semisolid waste may go into the sewage system. Contaminated or potentially infectious specimens, however, should be autoclaved before disposal, and any flammable waste, including empty, used specimen containers, should be incinerated if at all possible. Various categories of waste—potentially infectious material, glass, flammable and other solid waste—should be placed in separate containers lined with plastic bags so that cleaning people need not handle any of this material directly.

Potentially infectious waste must be handled with particular care. A separate container lined with a disposable, autoclave-resistant bag should be conveniently located for each employee dealing with such material. The bag should be taken from the container, closed, and autoclaved before being discarded.

If caustic or volatile materials are necessary for your lab procedures, keep only minimal quantities, and have a predetermined cleanup procedure to be followed in the case of a spill or a broken container. Cleanup materials should be segregated and clearly marked, and their disposal handled like that of comparable materials. Liquid or acid waste should be neutralized before putting it into the sewage system, and volatile waste should be evaporated in a suitable setting—a hood with a nonsparking exhaust fan is best. Liquid reagents or solvents containing cyanate must be significantly diluted before disposal in the sewage system, since high concentrations react chemically with copper piping to form explosive compounds that even a simple impact can detonate.

A SAFETY PROGRAM

Safety in the lab and office starts with the staff. Employees must appreciate the potential hazards they face so they can take steps to avoid injury. Prevention must thus start with education.

Another important part is a safety manual that details policies and safety practice. This should include designation of eating, drinking, and smoking areas, appropriate protective clothing and equipment, proscribed high-risk practices such as mouth pipetting, appropriate cleanup procedures for chemical spills, proper disposal of hazardous material, and any other potentially dangerous aspect of the practice.

A safety program should include the provision of certain equipment: Fire extinguishers, a fire blanket, an eye-wash fountain, and materials to neutralize spills of strong acids or caustic chemicals before cleanup are elements of a good program.

In both large and small laboratory settings, one person should be responsible for overseeing the safety program. This includes identifying new, potentially hazardous conditions, organizing safety drills, teaching others the proper use of firefighting equipment, and making periodic safety audits. Ideally, someone from another part of the office or an invited consultant should do these audits to spot potentially hazardous areas or practices—because people working in an area tend to get used to them.

It is not uncommon, for example, for someone using organic solvents to be insensitive to the high concentration of vapor in the air while any outsider notices it immediately. Similarly, an outsider may quickly see a potential electrical hazard, such as too many lines tying in to a single outlet or a wire stretched so that it's getting frayed.

Safety audits have both practical and legal liability value. Their results and any corrective action should be documented. This way, if accidents happen—and they will—the potential for tort liability damages can be minimized by demonstrating a climate of safe laboratory practice (Chapter 7).

GENERAL REFERENCES

1. Bond RG, Michaelson GS, DeRoos RL: *Environmental Health and Safety in Health Care Facilities*. New York, MacMillan, 1973.

2. Hartree E, Booth V: Safety in biological laboratories. *Biochem Soc Spec Publ* No. 5, 1977.

3. Steere NV: Safety management in the clinical laboratory, in Lundberg GD (ed): *Managing the Patient-Focused Laboratory*. Oradell, NJ, Medical Economics, 1975.

12

Hematology testing

In this chapter and the three succeeding ones, we will deal with testing in specific disciplines—hematology, chemistry, microbiology, and urinalysis. This classification may appear arbitrary from the office practitioner's perspective, but it is consistent with divisions in a hospital laboratory. Hematology tests fall into several categories that we will discuss separately: hemoglobin/hematocrit, white blood cell and differential counts, sedimentation rate, and coagulation tests. A list of hematology systems appears in Appendix 1.

HEMOGLOBIN/HEMATOCRIT

Recommended tests

We recommend the microhematocrit unless hemoglobin is measured as a by-product of a white cell count or as part of a chemistry system that does a variety of tests (Table 12-1).

Skill level required

Personnel with minimal on-the-job training can perform these tests.

Equipment

The microhematocrit requires a microhematocrit centrifuge and reader, which are single-purpose instruments that cannot be

Hemoglobin/hematocrit tests

Recommended tests
Microhematocrit
Hemoglobin as part of electronic WBC count
Hemoglobin measured in dry chemistry system

Skill level
Office assistant with on-the-job training

Equipment
Microhematocrit centrifuge with reader, or
Hemoglobin/WBC instrument, or
Dry chemistry system

Reagent stability
Long

Sources of error
Poor sample collection
Inadequate mixing of blood
Microhematocrit centrifuge speed too slow
Inadequate centrifugation time
Paralax error in reading
Pipetting error in hemoglobin procedure
Miscalibrated hemoglobinometer

Quality control
Check microhematocrit speed periodically
Measure constant packing time periodically
Check timer accuracy periodically
Use standards and controls for hemoglobin
Proficiency testing surveys

used for other centrifuging tasks. The centrifuge must have a reproducible speed and an accurate timer.

A filter colorimeter is necessary to measure hemoglobin. It can also be done with some of the cell-counting systems that contain a colorimeter, the Ames Seralyzer, dry reagent strip analyzer, or the Eastman Kodak Ektachem, dry slide analyzer.

Reagents and stability

The microhematocrit does not require chemical reagents. Reagents for hemoglobin determinations come in tablet or liquid form and are generally stable for a long time. The colorimeter's calibration must be periodically checked with a standard cyanmethemoglobin solution.

Sources of error

In measuring hematocrit, the most common errors are the technician's failure to mix the blood before filling the microhematocrit capillary tube, failure to centrifuge for the proper time, and viewing the microhematocrit tube from an angle causing a paralax error; the microhematocrit centrifuge may also fail to operate at the proper speed. A survey of physicians' office laboratories found that one popular brand of microhematocrit centrifuges operated at a speed lower than that specified by the manufacturer and gave hematocrit results that were too high. The major sources of error in the hemoglobin test are inaccurate pipetting of the blood, inadequate mixing of the blood before pipetting, and incorrect calibration of the colorimeter.

Quality-control requirements

The microhematocrit centrifuge should be tested monthly to make sure that it is running at the proper speed. The best way is to perform a microhematocrit test, centrifuge the blood for two minutes, take a reading, centrifuge again for one minute, take another reading, and repeat the last two steps until there is no change in the readings. This is known as the constant packing time, and these results should be recorded (Figure 12-1). The timer should also be checked for accuracy at monthly intervals.

A solution of known hemoglobin content such as a cyanmethemoglobin standard should be run each day that hemoglobin testing is performed. These standards are expensive, and unless a high volume of testing is done, this is an uneconomical procedure. An alternate approach involves analyzing a split specimen by the office lab and a reference lab.

Expected precision

Hemoglobin values in the normal range can be expected to be within ± 6% of the actual value 95% of the time. Hematocrit values in the normal range, as determined by the microhematocrit centrifuge method, can be expected to be within ± 6% of the actual value 95% of the time.

Quality control chart for hematology

Date	Technologist	Hematocrit control values			Reference/office lab results			Centrifuge speed/month	Centrifuge time from curve	Comments/problems
		1st run	+ 1 min	+ 2 min	HCT (+/−3%)	Hb (+/−0.5%)	WBC (+/−10%)			

This chart shows documentation of the constant packing time of the microhematocrit and comparisons of the office results for hematocrit, hemoglobin, and white cell count with those of the reference laboratory. Acceptable performance standards are shown along with a space for comments about problems encountered and action taken.

WHITE BLOOD CELL COUNT

Recommended tests

This test can be performed manually with a hemocytometer or electronic cell counter (Table 12-2). The hemocytometer is relatively inexpensive, but it is slower, requires a higher level of skill to perform, and is significantly less accurate than the electronic blood cell counter.

Skill level required

Someone without formal medical technology training can perform white cell counts by either method, but both require some skill and familiarity with how they work. The manual method requires attention to detail, manual dexterity in making the blood dilutions, and familiarity with the hemocytometer and the microscope.

Equipment

One or more hemocytometers are necessary for the manual method. Counting is done using a microscope with adequate light source. A pipetting-dilution system is necessary to make the dilutions. The simplest system is the Unopette from Becton Dickinson; it uses an accurate capillary pipette and a prefilled diluent container.

Several manufacturers produce automated cell counters. Most work on the principle that a blood cell passing through a small aperture in which an electric current is also passing causes a change in conductivity that the instrument can sense. The major differences between these instruments are related to how much adjustment the operator can make and which specific diluting systems must be used. For the office setting where someone without extensive medical technology training is likely to perform the test, we recommend an instrument that needs few operator adjustments and is not restricted to specific diluting systems. It should also have a method of flushing the counting aperture between cell counts.

A novel method for combined hematocrit and whole blood cell counting, the Clay Adams QBC, measures the hematocrit (packed red cell volume), leukocrit (packed white cell volume), and the plateletcrit (packed platelet volume). It also differentiates granulocytic from nongranulocytic white cells.

White blood count tests

Recommended test
Electronic WBC counting

Skill level
Office assistant with on-the-job training
Manual method requires greater skill

Equipment
Electronic blood cell counter, or
Hemocytometer, microscope
Capillary tube diluting system (Unopette)

Reagent stability
Long

Sources of error
Poor sample collection
Inadequate blood mixing
Inadequate pipetting
Counting chamber errors
Contaminated dilution fluid
Plugged electronic counter aperture
Miscalibration

Quality control
Duplicate counting using two chambers or two electronic counts
Weekly counts sent in parallel to another laboratory
Diluting fluid counts for background count
Proficiency testing surveys

Reagent stability

The diluting fluid, the only reagent used in this test, is relatively simple and stable for a long time.

Sources of error

- Tissue fluid will mix with the blood if a finger-stick specimen is taken without freely flowing blood;
- Inadequately mixing the venipuncture tube before pipetting the specimen;
- Inadequately filling the capillary pipette during the dilution stage;

- Incorrectly using the counting chamber;
- Using contaminated diluting fluid with the electronic cell counter;
- Not clearing a plugged aperture in the electronic instrument;
- Miscalibrating the electronic instrument.

Quality-control requirements

Duplicate counts for both manual and automated systems are desirable, and they should be done with two separate dilutions for greatest assurance of accuracy. These counts should agree closely. Once a week, we recommend sending a portion of a specimen that your laboratory has tested to a nearby reference laboratory and comparing the results. Periodically—once a week for the automated system and once a month for the manual system—you should perform a count on the diluting fluid itself. This is a background count to look for contaminants.

Your laboratory should also subscribe to one of several proficiency testing services that periodically send unknown samples for analysis. All personnel who will perform cell counts should receive some training from an experienced, thoroughly trained medical technologist.

Expected precision

With the hemocytometer, white cell counts in the normal range can be expected to be within $\pm 25\%$ of the actual value 95% of the time. With an electronic cell counter, values in the normal range should be within $\pm 6\%$ of the actual value 95% of the time.

PLATELET COUNTS

Recommended tests

Platelet counts are performed in the same way as white cell counts but require a greater level of skill. Although automated electronic instruments are available, they are generally dedicated instruments that are not used for white cell counts. Before platelets can be counted electronically, they must be concentrated with a special centrifuge and a red cell count done. Because of these complications and unless your practice is predominantly hematology or oncology, it is preferable to test platelet concentration

Platelet counts

Recommended test
  Bleeding time
Skill level
  Office assistant with on-the-job training
Equipment
  Spring-loaded bleeding time knife (Simplate II)
  Blood pressure cuff
  Stopwatch
Sources of error
  Excessive pressure on Simplate
  Inaccurate timing
  Patient's use of aspirin

---

and function by doing a bleeding time test (Table 12-3). General Diagnostics manufactures a spring-loaded device, the Simplate II, that makes a reproducible incision on the forearm for performing a standardized Ivy bleeding time.

BLOOD SMEAR EXAMINATION AND DIFFERENTIAL WHITE CELL COUNT

Recommended tests

Preparing and examining a blood smear require training, experience, and continued reinforcement; and unless a trained medical technologist is available, this test should be sent to a hospital or independent laboratory. If this is not feasible, a simplified differential count that distinguishes segmented neutrophils from all other white cells can be performed (Table 12-4). In this situation, a duplicate sample should be sent to a qualified laboratory for confirmation.

Skill level required

Knowledgeable examination of a blood smear requires training as a medical technologist and continued practice to maintain proficiency; not even many physicians are proficient in this procedure. A nontechnologist can be trained to do a modified differential count that distinguishes segmented neutrophils from all other white cells. A qualified medical technologist should do the training, which must include careful instruction in how to prepare the peripheral blood smear—a vital element in the examination. The smear must be scanned in a standardized pattern[1] because the cells are not evenly distributed on the slide (Figure 12-2). There should be ongoing communication between the reference laboratory and the office staff with regard to adequate smear preparation.

Equipment

A good microscope with oil immersion lens and a good light is essential for examining peripheral blood smears, and a mechanical or electronic differential counting enumerator should also be available. This avoids the tedious job of tallying the cells on a piece of paper and counting or calculating the percentages. A rack or other device for staining the slides is necessary if this will also be done in the office.

TABLE 12-4

Differential cell counts

Recommended tests
  Abbreviated neutrophil/nonneutrophil count

Skill level
  Well-trained office assistant
  Medical technologist for complete differential counts

Equipment
  Good microscope with oil immersion lens and good light
  Staining rack
  Cell counting enumerator

Reagent stability
  Long

Sources of error
  Poorly made blood smear
  Inadequate training or experience

Quality control
  Examination of duplicate slide by a qualified technologist
  Proficiency testing survey

How to scan a blood smear in a differential white cell count

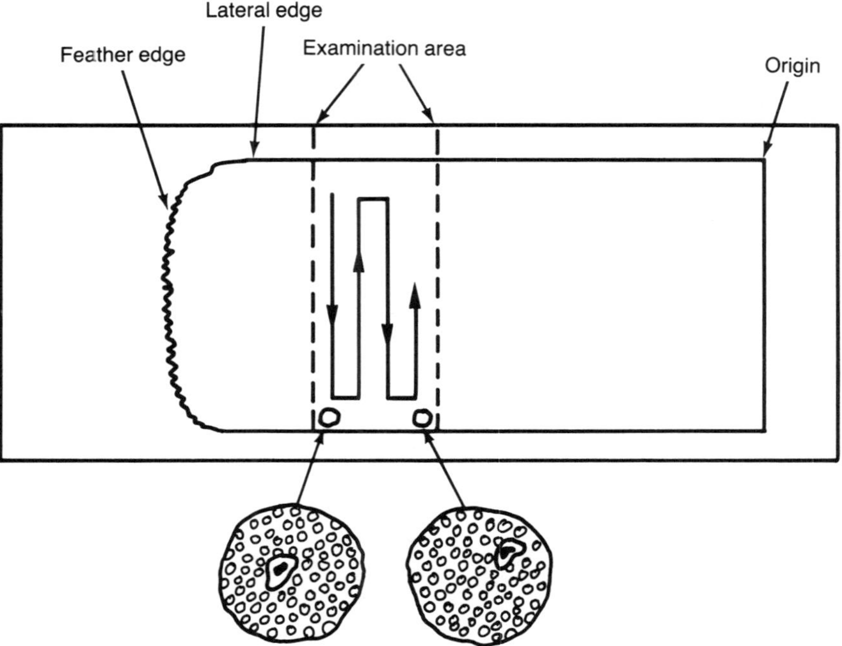

The figure at the bottom is a diagram of the distribution of cells in acceptable counting areas.

Reagents and stability

Prepared Wright's stain and methanol for fixing the slide and cleaning immersion oil off of the slide and microscope lenses is also necessary. All of these reagents are quite stable.

Sources of error

The major sources of error are related to the individual's inexperience in preparing the smears, staining the slides, or examining them. Not even a well-qualified technologist can read smears that are too thick—a common problem.

Quality-control requirements

Unless you have a well-qualified medical technologist to do these tests, it is best to send tubes of blood or blood smears to a hospital or independent laboratory. QC includes continued feedback from that laboratory about the adequacy of specimens.

Analyzing blood smears cannot be subjected to the statistical approach applied to cell counting and hemoglobin determination. It is particularly important to maintain the quality of the stain, especially where one batch of stain must be used for a long time because of low demand. The analyst must also have atlases or files of unusual findings for ready reference, and the physician must be available to consult about unusual or unexpected results.

It may be worthwhile to have the hospital laboratory reevaluate the slides and then to plot both sets of results for an evaluation of bias (Figure 12-3). A consulting hematologist should look at slides of concern or of unusual interest as part of the validation process and for the operators' continued education. Blood smear evaluation should include an estimate of the platelet count. Since this is an interpretative test involving the qualitative evaluation of the cells seen, the stained slide should be kept and filed in a way to allow easy retrieval should review become necessary.

Expected accuracy

In a 100-cell differential, the determined values can be expected to be within ± 20% of the actual proportion of neutrophilic leukocytes.[2] The range of error is less if more cells are counted or if the percentage of neutrophils is increased.

SEDIMENTATION RATE

A nonspecific indicator of increased acute phase proteins, the sedimentation rate is elevated in a variety of inflammatory conditions. The measurement is useful in several settings, however. In the pediatric age group, it indicates acute infection and is particularly helpful with small infants, where it is said to be more sensitive and more specific than the leukocyte count. In adults, it indicates rheumatic disease, with the rate falling in response to effective therapy.

Quality control for differential white counts

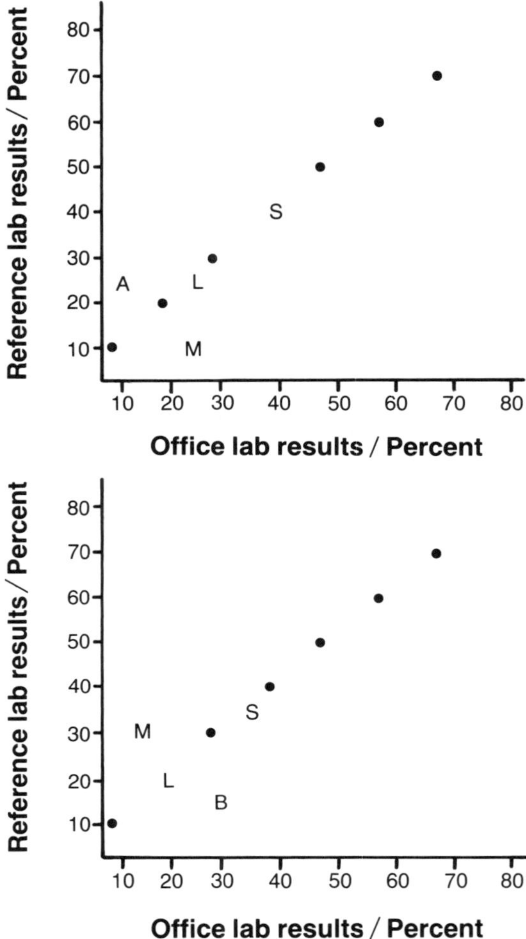

This method compares results from the office laboratory with those on the same blood smears processed in a reference laboratory. The plotted points are calculated by determining the average percent of each cell type as determined in each laboratory. In the examples shown here, there is apparently agreement on the percent of segmented neutrophils (S) and lymphocytes (L), but in the top panel, the office lab is apparently overestimating the number of monocytes (M) and underestimating the number of atypical lymphocytes (A). In the bottom panel there is an apparent confusion between monocytes (M) and segmented neutrophil band forms (B).

Recommended tests

The recommended method depends to some extent upon how the test will be used (Table 12-5). If it is to detect infection in children, the method should not be too sensitive in differentiating normal from abnormal. When the 200-mm Westergren tube is used, slightly to moderately abnormal values are found in some healthy individuals. This is because this particular method is especially sensitive to slight changes in red cell shape and mild degrees of anemia.

If the test is used for following patients with rheumatic disease, however, the long Westergren tube is preferred because differences in the highly abnormal range can be distinguished from one another; sensitivity in the high range is diminished with the shorter Wintrobe 100 millimeter tube. A compromise is the use of the capillary tube zeta sedimentation ratio (ZSR) method,[3] which has good sensitivity at both the high and low sedimentation ranges.

Another consideration in choosing a method is the length of time it takes to do the test. Blood must stand in the tube exactly 60 minutes before it is read in both the Wintrobe and Westergren methods. The ZSR is completed in three minutes. Of the three, the Westergren is the most complex, requiring a dilution of the blood sample with sodium citrate before drawing it up into the tube; the tube is also more difficult to fill. Newer self-filling disposable tubes have made these chores simpler, however.

If your practice is adult oriented and the sedimentation rate is used to assess rheumatoid disease, we recommend the Westergren method using disposable self-filling tubes. You might want to investigate the ZSR if your practice involves adults and children, if the test volume justifies a significant financial investment, and if the sedimentation rate is used both to assess rheumatoid disease and detect acute inflammatory disease.

Skill level required

Someone with minimal background in medical technology can easily learn the techniques of any of the three methods.

Equipment

Both the Wintrobe and Westergren methods require a special rack to hold the tubes vertical. A timer for exactly timing the 60 minutes is also necessary. The ZSR requires a special instrument

Sedimentation rate

Recommended tests
 For adult practice—Westergren ESR method
 For pediatric/adult practice—Zeta Sedimentation Rate (ZSR)
Skill level
 Office assistant with on-the-job training
Equipment
 Westergren disposable tubes with self-filling and dilution vial features, and
tube rack
 60-minute timer
 ZSR centrifuge and microhematocrit centrifuge with reader
 Aliquot mixer
Reagent stability
 Long
Sources of error
 Nonlevel ESR rack
 Vibration
 Poorly controlled room temperature
 Anemia or polycythemia
 Abnormal RBC size or shape
 Inaccurate pipetting
 Inadequate mixing
 Testing delay after obtaining blood sample
Quality control
 Parallel testing of a sample in another laboratory

---

with reader. This is a slow-speed centrifuge that holds the capillary tubes in a vertical position rotating first in one direction, then the reverse. The ZSR method also requires doing a microhematocrit (with its own centrifuge and reader) on the tube after reading the sedimentation. It is handy to have an aliquot mixer because the blood sample should be mixed thoroughly for two minutes before taking a sample and again for two minutes if it is diluted with sodium citrate.

Reagents and stability

Blood must be collected in EDTA for all three methods, and it must be diluted with sodium citrate with the Westergren method.

These reagents are all stable for a long time.

Sources of error

- The rack holding the tubes must be absolutely level. Tilting them by only three degrees will cause a 30% increase in the ESR. The rack must therefore have a leveling indicator, and the feet should be adjustable. Some of the disposable self-filling systems come with a level plastic rack.
- Vibration elevates the sedimentation rate.
- The test is sensitive to ambient temperature; extremes of heat or cold will cause errors.
- Anemia and polycythemia have a significant effect on the Westergren and Wintrobe methods. There are correction tables to correct for anemia with the Westergren. These tables are not valid for the Wintrobe method. The ZSR method is self-correcting for anemia.
- Variations in cell size and shape cause changes unrelated to the change in proteins.
- Inaccurate specimen diluting or pipetting causes errors. Pipetting should never be done by mouth.
- Inadequate mixing of the specimen before diluting or filling the tube.
- Delay in testing a specimen; the test should be run within several hours of collection.

Quality-control requirements

Traditional QC methods such as running a known specimen at the same time as the unknown patient's specimen are not applicable to this test. Periodically, a sample should be split, with half being run in your laboratory and half being sent to a reference laboratory that uses the same method. Make sure that the test is run promptly in the outside laboratory, because a significant time delay causes varying results.

Expected precision

There are no data for the expected precision of this test, but it is reasonable to expect that with the Westergren method, the determined value should be within ± 3 mm of the actual value 95% of the time. Using the ZSR, the determined value should be within ± 2.5% of the actual value 95% of the time.

COAGULATION TESTS

Coagulation tests that might be performed in the doctor's office fall into two categories: those to detect or diagnose abnormal bleeding disorders and those to monitor and control anticoagulant therapy. The prothrombin time (PT) test for monitoring coumarin therapy is sometimes performed in doctors' office laboratories (Table 12-6). The decision about whether or not to do this test depends on several factors. Its reagents are rather expensive, and once opened and reconstituted, they are stable only a few hours. Although manual PT methods test are available, an automated instrument is much more accurate. But it may be prohibitively expensive, particularly if only occasionally needed.

On the other hand, specimens for PT tests are unstable and cannot be mailed, so you may have to do these tests in your office if there's no reference laboratory nearby.

Recommended methods

Prothrombin time tests can be performed manually, using a test tube, water bath, a good light, and a stopwatch, but it is technically exacting, requiring accurate temperature control, precise timing, and reproducible and consistent agitation. This procedure is much more accurate with one of the mechanical coagulation instruments. In one survey of doctors' office laboratories, about 25% were performing PT tests, and more than half of these used instruments.

We recommend an automated coagulation instrument that uses an optical or electrical end-point. Prothrombin results are influenced by many factors including the choice of instrument and reagent system. If you are practicing at a hospital where its laboratory will perform PTs on your patients, it is very helpful to use the same type of instrument and reagent system in your office for comparability.

Skill level required

Manual PT tests require a high degree of manual dexterity and theoretical understanding of the test and its sources of error, and should be used only by a trained medical technologist. The automated procedure takes less education and experience because many of the critical factors in performing the test are under the instrument's control.

TABLE 12-6

Coagulation tests

Recommended test
Automated prothrombin time
Skill level
Office assistant with on-the-job training
Equipment
Automated coagulation instrument with accurate heater and timer
Pipettes
Reagent stability
Long for unopened reagent and control materials; refrigeration required
One day in refrigerator after opening
Specimen should be tested within six hours
Sources of error
Poor temperature control
Inaccurate timing
Poor pH control of water to reconstitute thromboplastin or control
Reagent or control kept too long after reconstitution
Specimen not tested promptly
Unclear instrument
Quality control
Use two control plasma specimens daily
Measure and record instrument temperature daily
Check timer accuracy monthly
Measure and record refrigerator temperature daily
Check pH of water for reconstituting reagent and control

Equipment

The instrument is a self-contained unit with compartments for preheating the specimen and reagents, a heated well for performing the test, a timer, and a detection system for sensing the clot. The detection system must be compatible with the reagents that are to be used. Opaque reagent systems cannot be used with optical detectors.

Reagent stability

Both the control materials and thromboplastin are labile and must be kept under refrigeration before and after reconstitution. Once reconstituted, they can be used only for one day.

Factors that contribute to erroneous results

Falsely low values	Falsely high values
Microhematocrit	
1. Viewing the tube from an angle causing a parallax error	1. Viewing the tube from an angle causing a parallax error
2. Inadequately mixing blood before filling the capillary tube and drawing the specimen from the plasma-rich area at the top of the tube	2. Including the buffy coat in reading the red cell volume
3. Inadequately filling the collection tube so that the anticoagulant over dilutes the blood sample	3. Inadequately mixing the blood before filling the capillary tube and drawing the specimen from the cell-rich area at the bottom of the tube
4. Reading the hematocrit a long time after the specimen has been spun	4. Failure of the centrifuge to operate at the proper speed or for enough time resulting in less than maximal packing of the red blood cells
5. Improper centrifugation timing	5. Increased plasma trapping because of unusually shaped cells such as macrocytes, sickle cells, and poikilocytes
	6. Using EDTA-anticoagulated blood that has been stored for more than 24 hours
White cell count	
1. Finger is squeezed to obtain a sample resulting in excess tissue fluid mixing with the blood	1. In an agitated patient the WBC may be elevated as a result of a stress reaction
2. Inadequately mixing blood before drawing the sample from the venipuncture tube	2. Inadequately mixing blood before drawing the blood from the venipuncture tube
3. Inadequately filling the capillary pipette in a manual count	3. Counting a chamber that has been filled excessively with solution overflowing the counting area in a count
4. Underfilling the counting chamber	4. Using contaminated diluting fluid with an electronic cell counter
5. Bubbles in the counting chamber	5. Miscalibrating an electronic counting instrument
6. A plugged aperture in the electronic cell counter	
7. Miscalibrating an electronic counting instrument	

Hemoglobin

Falsely low values	Falsely high values
1. Inadequately mixing blood before drawing the sample from the plasma-rich area at the top of the tube	1. Inadequately mixing blood before drawing the sample from the cell-rich area at the bottom of the tube
2. Pipetting less than standard volume	2. Pipetting more than standard volume
3. Incorrectly calibrating the colorimeter	3. Incorrectly calibrating the colorimeter

Erythrocyte sedimentation rate

Falsely low values	Falsely high values
1. Microcytic red blood cells settle slower than normocytic cells and cause a lower ESR	1. Tilting of the sedimentation tube as little as 3 degrees will cause a 30% increase in the ESR
2. Diluting the specimen with too much anticoagulant	2. Vibrations
3. Inadequately mixing sample before diluting or filling tube	3. Anemia (ZSR is self correcting)
4. Polycythemia	4. Room temperature above 25 C.
5. Excessive delay between collecting the sample and processing the test	5. Macrocytic red cells settle faster than normocytic cells and may elevate the ESR (correction tables are available)
6. Misshaped red blood cells such as sickle cells or spherocytes	

Reticulocyte count

Falsely low values	Falsely high values
1. Reticulocytes in blood that has a high concentration of glucose do not take up the reticulocyte stain	1. Failure to correct the count for anemia
2. Insufficiently mixing the sample	2. Counting cells with refractile artifacts as reticulocytes
	3. Insufficiently mixing the sample
	4. Counting other red cell inclusions as reticulum including Howell-Jolly bodies, Heinz bodies, and Pappenheimer bodies

continued

Falsely low values	Falsely high values
Sickle cell screen	
1. Until age 3 months an affected child's blood may not have a high enough concentration of hemoglobin S to give a positive reaction (the infant's red cells contain primarily fetal hemoglobin)	1. Elevated protein (as in multiple myeloma) will cause floculation of the solution producing an apparent positive result
2. Other hemoglobinopathies may give a positive result	
3. Insufficient blood sample, as from a patient with a hematocrit of less than 20	
4. Testing of old, unrefrigerated blood	
5. Recent transfusion	
6. Inactive reagent, as from using a test kit after the expiration date	
Prothrombin time	
1. Rapidly agitating the specimen during the clotting period	1. Acid or alkaline water used to reconstitute control plasma or thromboplastin
2. Inaccurately timing the clotting reaction	2. Inaccurately timing the clotting reaction
3. Inadequate temperature control during clotting	3. Inadequate temperature control during clotting
4. Dirty test tube or electrical sensing probe	4. Dirty test tube or electrical sensing probe

Sources of error

Temperature must be controlled within 0.1 C, and timing should be accurate within one second. Too fast agitation during the clotting period can accelerate the reaction, so it should be constant and reproducible. The reaction can be inhibited if the pH of the water used to reconstitute the thromboplastin or control plasma is too acid or too alkaline. Test tubes must be scrupulously clean and free of scratches. The instrument's electrical sensing probe must be clean and without traces of fibrin or thromboplastin. The specimen should be refrigerated if it is not tested promptly, and if possible, the plasma should be separated and removed from red cells within two hours of venipuncture. It should be stored in a capped tube no longer than six hours before testing.

Quality-control requirements[4]

Each day that the PT test is run, two control plasmas, one normal and one abnormal, should be run. Their values should be satisfactory before doing patient tests. Because the reaction is extremely temperature sensitive, the incubator's temperature should be measured and recorded daily. And because thermometers can vary in their accuracy, the thermometer used for this important check should be calibrated against a certified thermometer in the hospital laboratory. The refrigerator temperature should also be measured and recorded daily because reagents and controls must be refrigerated for a long time. The instrument timer should be periodically checked against a standard timer. The simplest way to do this is to compare it with the telephone time message for a minute or two. The water used to reconstitute control plasma and thromboplastin should be checked for pH neutrality.

Expected precision

Among laboratories tested in the College of American Pathologists proficiency survey, the CV for the PT test is about 8%.[2] In a recent survey of doctors' office laboratories, the CV ranged from 17% to 20%.[5] Stating this in another way, the answers from office laboratories sent an unknown specimen whose PT was 28 seconds, ranged from 18 to 45 seconds; the responses for a specimen with a PT of 12 seconds ranged from 7 to 17 seconds. On a day-to-day basis, the CV within the laboratory should be about 4% for a normal control plasma and about 5% for an abnormal control plasma.

Table 12-7 outlines common factors that can contribute to erroneous results.

REFERENCES

1. Fischer PM, Addison LA, Curtis P, et al: *The Office Laboratory.* Norwalk, Conn, Appleton-Century-Crofts, 1983.

2. Elevitch FR, Noce PS: Data Recap 1970-1980. Skokie, Ill, College of American Pathologists, 1981.

3. Bull BS: Clinical and laboratory implications of present ESR methodology. *Clin Lab Haemat* 1981;3:283-298.

4. Miale JB, *Laboratory Medicine Hematology*, ed 6. St. Louis, CV Mosby, 1982, pp 385-387.

5. Personal communication, Bureau of Laboratories, Commonwealth of Pennsylvania Department of Health.

13

Chemistry testing

Recent advances in technology have made a wide variety of chemistry tests available for the office laboratory. In the past, performing these analyses called for several exacting steps: accurately pipetting serum and reagents into test tubes, incubating them for precise times, and reading a colorimeter after standardization with a solution of known concentration. Results had to be mathematically calculated with a formula that related the instrument readings of the standards and unknown specimen to their concentrations.

Today's microprocessor-controlled instruments have taken much of the drudgery out of these manual procedures. Instrument and reagent stability have developed to the point where standardization is required only once a day—or even less. Wavelength and calibration factors can be set automatically, as can incubations and multiple readings.

In some systems, the user merely touches a sensor to indicate the proper test. In others, an optical code or magnetic strip in the reagent set tells the instrument which test to do. Automatic pipetting devices have also greatly simplified chemistry testing and made the results more accurate. A list of chemistry systems appears in Appendix 1.

RECOMMENDED SYSTEMS

The ideal chemistry system requires a minimum of operator intervention. It should include these automatic features: pipetting devices, photometer settings, temperature regulation, incubation timing and reading of results at the right times during incubation, and calculation of results from previously set standards. All of these are in fact available in presently marketed test systems.

The physician's office laboratory today has a wide array of choices. They range from simple meters that read color intensity in the reaction tube to fully automated test systems. The simplest manual test-tube system requires the technician to blank and calibrate the photometer for a specific assay, aspirate a measured amount of serum specimen with a pipette, add it to a test tube containing a measured amount of a reagent, mix it, incubate it for an accurately timed interval, and read the resulting color intensity with a photometer. An enzyme test requires several timed readings of the changing color reaction.

In such manual systems, variance can be introduced at several steps. They demand accurate pipetting, mixing, temperature control, and timing. A slip-up anywhere along the line can contribute to analytic error. Incorrectly setting the photometer wavelength, omitting the blanking step, or failing to check for a shift in the photometer's calibration can also cause errors.

Semiautomated and fully automated chemistry test systems have greatly decreased variance and the time and number of steps in these analyses. Several sophisticated, microprocessor-controlled, test-tube systems provide accurate pipetting devices, automatic wavelength selection, highly stable electronics that require infrequent calibration, internal incubators with automatic timing devices, multiple readings for enzyme determinations, and automatic calculation and printing of test results. Prepackaged reagents usually come with the systems.

Still another innovation is dry reagent testing, a technology that promises to change chemistry testing in all sizes of laboratories. In one system (the Ames Seralyzer), the user dilutes serum with water and then applies measured specimen to a test strip similar to a urine dipstick. Incubation starts when the stick is inserted in the instrument, then one or more timed readings are made, and the result is calculated and displayed. These tests are available now: aspartate aminotranferase (AST, SGOT), BUN, cholesterol, creatine kinase (CK), creatinine, glucose, hemoglobin, lactate dehydrogenase (LD, LDH), potassium, theophylline, total bilirubin, triglycerides, and uric acid. Soon to come are alanine aminotransferase (ALT, SGPT), amylase, and gamma glutamlytransferase (GGT).

Other new integrated test systems offer a similar scope of tests. One of them (the Reflotron from Boehringer Mannheim Diagnostics [BMD]) uses an unmeasured whole blood sample. Putting the blood on the strip starts a process that extracts plasma and collects it in a reservoir. Inserting the strip in the instrument puts the attached reagent packet into contact with the plasma reservoir, drawing the plasma into the dry reagent packet by capillary action, and initiating the analytic reaction. The instrument reads timing, wavelength, and calibration information from a strip of magnetic tape that is an integral component of the reagent stick.

Several new systems use film (much like photographic film) that is impregnated with reagents. In one of these (the Kodak DT60), the instrument places undiluted serum or plasma on the film, which also carries the fully automated testing sequence with calibration and wavelength information as a bar code.

Skill level required

With semiautomated systems, no formal medical technology training is required. The operator needs a good degree of manual dexterity, but on-the-job training from the company representative is enough to learn how to operate the system and do individual tests. When new people are hired, it is best to have the company representative train them, too.

Equipment

In the doctor's office laboratory with minimally trained technical help, the ideal instrument is simple to operate and has few manual steps. It should be an integrated system with a pipetting device, incubator, colorimeter, and reagents. Automated wavelength selection, calibration, temperature control, and timing are also desirable. We recommend buying from a large, well-known, well-established company that can continue to support its products; Abbott, Ames, Baker, BMD, Kodak, and Mallinckrodt all offer integrated chemistry systems. Ames and BMD also manufacture glucose monitoring systems in which whole blood is applied to a test strip. They require manual timing and wiping or washing the blood off the strip before measuring the reaction in the colorimeter. A list of the systems and vendor addresses and phone numbers can be found in the Appendix.

Reagents and stability

Reagents are available in several forms. Reagent strips, packaged much like urine dipsticks, are relatively stable at room temperature as long as the container is tightly closed and protected from moisture.

In test-tube systems, reagents may be dry in packages, premeasured in test tubes, or dispensed from vials. Depending on the test and the system, the reagents may require room temperature storage, refrigeration, or freezing. Reagents for enzyme tests have a limited life and may require refrigeration.

Sources of error

Chemistry tests are subject to many sources of error, most of which can be minimized by good technique and rigid quality control (QC). Periodic standardization and running QC samples each time the test is performed minimizes errors and makes them more apparent when they do occur. We discuss these errors fully in Chapter 17, but a partial list includes pipetting errors, deteriorated reagents, instrument instability, improper standardization, improperly set wavelengths, dirty instruments, scratched or dirty test tubes, calculation errors, incorrect timing, incorrect incubation temperatures, clerical errors in recording results, and a mismatch of reagents and equipment.

Quality control

Clinical chemistry lends itself to effective QC better than most other areas of the laboratory. The accreditation rules for hospital and independent laboratories are very specific about QC requirements. At least two standards (calibrators) of different concentrations should be run each day that the test is performed unless the manufacturer indicates otherwise. Reagent inserts indicate the range of linearity for the test. Results outside of this range must be diluted and repeated to obtain correct results.

QC samples should be run, recorded, and charted each time a group of tests is performed. It is good practice to run them in two ranges. An expanded discussion of QC controls can be found in Chapter 17. The manufacturers' instructions describe preventive maintenance procedures, which should be performed exactly and recorded in a log. The QC and maintenance logs should also detail any problems and their solutions.

Heat blocks, water baths, and incubators should have thermometers whose temperatures must be recorded daily. Reagents are marked with expiration dates, and it is important to discard any that are outdated. Most reagents also have a finite life once the package is opened. It should be marked with an expiration date to assure that it is discarded at the proper time. A procedure manual containing current package inserts should be available—and you should be aware that manufacturers occasionally change package insert instructions without notifying their customers.

Expected precision

With semiautomated chemistry equipment, 95% of test results should be within ± 10% of the true value. Enzyme tests are somewhat less accurate; 95% of their results should be within ± 20% of the true value.

HOW TO EVALUATE CHEMISTRY SYSTEMS

With so many systems for chemistry testing available on the market, the options become overwhelming. This section will discuss some of the more desirable features. Unfortunately, no single system includes all of them, but by considering each feature, you should be in a better position to make an intelligent choice.

Scope of tests

The range of tests should be wide enough to include most of the clinically relevant tests you want to perform. It will probably include enzymatic procedures, electrolytes, and therapeutic drug monitoring.

Cost

Many factors influence the cost of doing a laboratory test. Besides the initial outlay for the instrument, you must consider maintenance and service costs, which generally run 10% to 15% of the purchase price. If the office must be remodeled to accommodate the equipment, this must also be considered part of the purchase cost. In a sense, a restricted range of tests also constitutes a cost because the alternative is to send it to another laboratory and lose income.

Reagent costs also go beyond the direct outlay. Efficiency in using the reagent will be directly related to its per-test cost. Some systems are quite wasteful in that once the reagent is reconstituted or opened, it must be used. True per-test cost is thus related to how many tests can be expected from each vial or bottle rather than the theoretical maximum number of tests that can be performed. If an instrument is quite stable in its calibration, it will not need frequent standardization, saving reagents and labor and also providing more patient tests per unit.

The same factors that relate to reagent cost are true of controls. Some are more efficiently packaged and more stable than others. In general, a multiparameter control material with a wide range of constituents cuts waste and cost. The best instrument and reagent systems have a wide range of linearity between instrument reading and concentration. If the range is too narrow, too many tests outside the range will have to be repeated, with added reagent and labor costs. Finally, storage must also be considered a cost factor: Some reagent systems are quite bulky, and some require refrigeration. More information about cost accounting can be found in Chapter 8.

Speed of testing

In the small laboratory, it is customary to do several tests for one patient, rather than a relatively large batch of identical tests for different patients. Thus a test system that allows easy switching between different tests, without recalibrations or extensive instrument or reagent changes, is desirable. It can also be an advantage to perform a test on whole blood, rather than having to centrifuge the specimen and separate serum. In larger group practice laboratories where specimens may accumulate over time or where serum is frequently required for reference lab tests, it may be important for the instrument to have the dual capability of analyzing either whole blood or serum specimens. Another plus is a system that takes a minimum of technologist's time.

Accuracy and precision

Today's technology often makes it possible to achieve accuracy and precision comparable to that achieved in hospital laboratories. In general, coefficients of variation (CVs) of 5% are achievable for most tests—even greater for some. Enzyme tests usually have a precision within 10% for one CV.

Quality control

Good quality control is the key to confidence in your laboratory work. Good instrument manuals including trouble-shooting guides are essential system features. Some advanced instruments can perform self-checks on their optical and electronic systems before measuring patient samples. And several manufacturers have considered including microprocessors that would check the acceptability of the QC sample before releasing patient data. This feature is not presently available, but in our opinion it would be highly desirable.

Pipetting

This manual skill is relatively easy to learn, but it does require a degree of manual dexterity and concentration, and it also adds to analysis time. There are some advantages to a system—such as dry chemistry—that does not require the specimen to be measured or has a wide tolerance for sample quantity. A system that does not require diluting the sample also eliminates a pipetting step.

Reagents

Reagent costs vary markedly depending on packaging and the type of chemistry involved. Premeasured, individually packaged reagents are generally preferable because they eliminate a measuring step, provide increased stability, and cut waste. Reagent storage may also be a problem because some take a lot of space, and some must be kept refrigerated or frozen.

Incubation

In one evaluation of an automated dry chemistry system,[1] most of the operator variance appeared to come from timing errors during incubation. Thus an instrument for the physician's office lab should automatically control incubation timing and temperature; automatic reading of the concentration after incubation is also desirable.

Calibration

Many chemistry tests have a nonlinear relationship between the analyte concentration and the instrument reading in a portion of the calibration curve, so it is desirable to calibrate at several concentrations. The calibrator should be usable in all chemistry calibrations and it should be handled as if it were a test sample, undergoing all the same processes. It should have long stability once it is opened or reconstituted—most today are stable for several weeks if the manufacturer's storage recommendations are followed.

Reading results

Because several different tests may be performed consecutively on a single patient, it is desirable for the instrument to recognize automatically each reagent pack or tube. In some systems, once the reagent pack has been identified, the instrument sets the reading parameters, measures the reaction, and calculates the results. Without this degree of automation, the less-experienced operator may easily forget to change settings between tests, thus producing erroneous results.

The photometer's optical system should be high quality with a narrow-band wavelength. Cheaper filter systems will produce readings that are less linear in their response to concentration differences and less specific in excluding interfering reactions. The system should be self-blanking so that it is unnecessary to set up a reagent or specimen blank tube; it should be capable of reading and calculating rate reactions for enzymatic reactions; and it should flag out-of-range results that are too high or too low for it to read. With the inexpensive microprocessors available today, we should also look for instruments that can calculate results from stored calibration information, as well as print patient identification information along with the results to avoid transcription errors and loss of data.

THERAPEUTIC DRUG TESTING

Dry chemistry reagent systems have made it possible to analyze a variety of drugs—specifically theophylline, phenytoin, and phenobarbital—in the physician's office laboratory. Several systems also measure potassium, which is monitored when digoxin, steroids, or antihypertensive agents are administered. Chapter 5 discusses the clinical aspects of therapeutic drug monitoring.

Skill level required

Personnel with on-the-job training in using dry chemistry systems can produce accurate, precise results if they have been properly oriented to potential sources of error. Of even greater importance is proper education about how the specimens must be drawn.

Equipment

The tests are performed on a dry chemistry system. Other necessary equipment is a centrifuge for separating plasma or serum if samples are prepared for shipment to reference laboratories.

Reagent stability

Dry chemistry reagents are stable for a long time, usually a year if the strips in the container are carefully kept dry and protected from excessive heat. The reagent containers have a desiccant in them to protect the strips against excessive humidity.

Sources of error

It is essential to operate the equipment properly, with the most important source of error being accurate timing of the reaction. Of even greater importance—and unrelated to the analytic technique itself—is the proper timing of specimen collection. Depending on the bioavailability of a drug and its absorption characteristics, there is a rise in blood concentration followed by a decrease to a trough level after the drug is ingested. The time of decrease is related to the drug's excretion, metabolic characteristics, and tissue binding. Most drugs are measured at their lowest or trough level, and if the specimen is drawn too soon, the value will be a falsely elevated. The time of drawing and the time of ingestion of the last dose should always be recorded and made part of the final report.

Quality control

In addition to the usual standardization and measurement of quality-control samples, record keeping is an essential part of therapeutic drug monitoring. As mentioned, this includes recording when the specimen was collected and when the last dose was ingested.

PHENOBARBITAL

When to sample

At least 18 days after starting or changing dosage. It is best to obtain a sample just before the next dose, but it can be drawn any time without causing a significant error. There is only a slight difference between peak and trough concentrations of phenobarbital because of its long half-life.

Pitfalls in the assay

Some analytical systems measure phenobarbital metabolites, which can cause a problem in patients with renal failure.

Pitfalls in interpretation

This drug is moderately bound to protein. If the serum albumin is markedly reduced, therapeutic and toxic effects can occur at lower concentrations.

Therapeutic and toxic ranges

Therapeutic: 15-30 μg/mL.
Toxic: >40 μg/mL; coma occurs at >90 mcg/mL.

PHENYTOIN

When to sample

At least five days after starting or changing the dosage. It is best to obtain a sample just before the next dose, but it can be drawn any time without causing a significant error. There is only a slight difference between peak and trough concentrations of phenytoin because of its long half-life.

Pitfalls in interpretation

This drug is markedly bound to protein. If the serum albumin is reduced, therapeutic and toxic effects can occur at lower concentrations.

Therapeutic and toxic ranges

Therapeutic: 10-20 μg/mL. Seizure control appears to be directly proportional to the optimum serum concentration.
Toxic: Nystagmus may occur at >20 μg/mL; ataxia is frequent at >30 μg/mL; lethargy occurs at >40 μg/mL.

THEOPHYLLINE

When to sample

At least two days after starting or changing the dosage. Anytime between doses; when long-acting preparations are used, there is little difference between peak and trough concentrations.

Pitfalls in interpretation

If the patient is receiving a nonsustained-action dose, sampling should occur two hours after the oral dose is given. If it is sampled later, the assay will underestimate potential toxicity of a dosage schedule.

Therapeutic and toxic ranges

Therapeutic: 10-20 μg/mL.
Toxic: At >25 μg/mL, 75% of patients show toxic effects.

REFERENCE
1. Clark PMS, Broughton PMS: Potential applications and pitfalls of dry reagent tests. An evaluation of the Ames Seralyzer. *Ann Clin Biochem* 1983;20:208-212.

GENERAL REFERENCE
Baer DM, Dito WR: *Interpretation of Therapeutic Drug Monitoring.* Chicago, American Society of Clinical Pathologists, 1981.

14

Microbiology testing

The amount of microbiology work done in the office laboratory will depend upon the size and type of practice. Few infections in outpatients are life-threatening, and most can be diagnosed with a handful of procedures. A list of microbiology test systems can be found in Appendix 1.

CULTURE PROCEDURES

About 90% of the microbiologic specimens in an office lab will be analyzed for urinary tract infections (UTIs), pharyngitis, or genital infections. Among the advantages of doing in-office cultures are the elimination of specimen transport problems, cost saving for the patient, and faster results. The disadvantages include the need to train and supervise personnel, the cost and other problems of buying supplies, increased space requirements, and implementing a quality-control program.

Recommended tests

The most common and easily performed procedures include throat and urine cultures, those for *Neisseria gonorrhoeae*, and microscopy for Gram stains and wet mounts (Table 14-1). Depending on the level of information desired, these procedures require a minimum of expertise and quality control. Other microbiology tests that demand more expertise and quality control should not

TABLE 14-1

Culture procedures

Recommended tests
Cultures for *N. gonorrhoeae*
Gram-stained smears
Throat cultures
Urine cultures
Wet mount preparations

Skill level needed
Office trained
 Inoculate cultures
 Gram-stain smears,
 Read cultures for bacterial growth
Medical technologist/technician
 Interpret Gram-stained smears and cultures

Equipment
Bacteriologic loops
Electric incinerator or alcohol lamp
Incubator
Microscope
Refrigerator

Reagent stability
Media are sensitive to dehydration and contamination
Reagents are sensitive to heat and contamination

Sources of error
Improperly collected and transported specimens
Inappropriate incubation
Misinterpreted results by inexperienced personnel
Unacceptable media and reagents

Quality control
Confirm results with experienced microbiologist
Monitor equipment temperature
Prepare and use a procedure manual
Test media and reagents with stock organisms

be performed in a routine office laboratory; they include susceptibility testing; identifying gram-negative bacilli; parasitology examinations; and cultures of stool, blood, and sputum.

The office laboratory can use a variety of routine culture methods and some new nonculture techniques for the presumptive identification of *N. gonorrhoeae*, *Streptococcus pyogenes*, and *Staphylococcus aureus*. The Gram stain, for example, is one of the best ways to diagnose infectious diseases, and can also serve as a check on the quality of the specimen and the culture results. The time necessary to gain microscopic interpretive expertise is well spent. Other simple procedures include slide agglutination and oxidase, catalase, coagulase, and bacitracin susceptibility tests.

The nonculture procedures now becoming available will eventually eliminate many of the older culture methods; they are faster and require less technical expertise. Among them are slide agglutination tests for the direct detection of bacterial antigens and a variety of methods to screen specimens for the presence of bacteria (see Chapter 15). Many of these tests are promising, but need more study before finally replacing the culture methods.

Skill level

Office and nursing personnel can easily learn techniques for Gram-staining smears and inoculating culture media. Interpreting the smears, culture results, and most biochemical tests, however, should be done by the physician or a trained medical technologist or technician.

Equipment

Major initial equipment costs are for a refrigerator, microscope, incubator, and electric incinerator or alcohol lamp. Other necessary purchases are for such miscellaneous supplies as microscope slides, bacteriologic loops, culture media, and reagents.

Reagent stability

Reagents used in a microbiology laboratory include stains, culture media, and materials for specific biochemical tests. Media should be examined when received for any signs of deterioration such as dehydration, contamination, or precipitated material.

Commercial media have a clearly marked package expiration date that varies with the type of medium. These dates should be strictly observed since deterioration significantly lowers growth and recovery rates. In general, media containing enrichments should be used within three months from the date of preparation. Tubed media without enrichments are stable from six months to a year.

Test reagents and stains are also labeled with an expiration date. Their stability, however, depends on storage conditions and packaging; failure to follow the manufacturer's instructions can make the date invalid.

Sources of error

There are two major causes of inappropriate culture results. First, if specimens are improperly collected, transported, or incubated, the infectious agent will fail to grow or normal flora will overcome it. Second, untrained personnel misinterpret culture and test results. We will discuss specific problems in Chapter 17.

Quality control

It is difficult to define the minimum quality-control (QC) procedures for an office microbiology laboratory. In general, they should include a good procedure manual; reagent and media QC with appropriate control organisms; monitoring equipment temperature; and participating in some type of proficiency testing program such as a commercial program or informal exchange of unknown organisms. All reagents and media should be labeled as to lot number, date of preparation, date of receipt, and expiration date. In addition, each shipment should be checked for sterility and adequate performance with stock cultures unless a local manufacturer prepares the media and the laboratory receives them on the same shipping day.

Stains and test reagents should be tested with stock organisms when they are put into service and thereafter at regular intervals or with each use. On some tests, QC serves as a visual example to aid in the interpretation and should be done with each test. The best QC procedure is the periodic review and confirmation of results with an experienced microbiologist.

Biohazardous waste can be handled by immersing the material in 5% bleach and then disposing of it with other material or by making arrangements with a reference laboratory for sterilization. Counter tops should be disinfected daily with a phenolic base disinfectant; personnel should wear laboratory coats and wash their hands often with an antiseptic soap.

Expected accuracy

Sensitivity, specificity, precision, and accuracy are difficult to determine for specific microbiology procedures. The recovery of bacterial isolates from a clinical specimen depends upon a number of variables: the host, the timing of the culture or test in relation to the stage of the infection, whether or not the patient is receiving an antimicrobial agent, and most important, the appropriate collection and handling of the specimen and the expertise of the personnel performing the tests.

MICROSCOPIC PROCEDURES

The direct microscopic examination of clinical specimens, either by Gram-stained smear or wet mount, is one of the most useful procedures for the rapid diagnosis of infectious diseases. It provides evidence for specimen quality and the organism or organisms responsible for the infection, and acts as a QC check on the culture results. In some specimens, finding many leukocytes and a few squamous epithelial cells on the Gram stain indicates a well-collected specimen.

Recommended tests

A Gram stain should be prepared on all specimens except throat specimens (Table 14-2). After staining, examine the smear under low power (10×) to assess the quality of the specimen. In general, an appropriate specimen (genital, sputum, or wound, for example) contains polymorphonuclear leukocytes (PMNs) and infrequent squamous epithelial cells (SECs). An adequate expectorated sputum specimen should show PMNs and fewer than 10 to 25 SECs per low-power field.

Next switch to the 100× objective, and assess the technical adequacy of the stain. Gram-positive organisms are dark-blue to purple; gram-negative organisms and PMN nuclei are pink to red. PMN color is the best control for undercolorization of the smear. Examine several areas and fields of the smear, noting the quantity, morphology, and Gram reaction of the organisms (Table 14-3). Look particularly for a predominant organism.

The saline wet mount is helpful for diagnosing vaginitis caused by *Trichomonas vaginalis*. Place a drop of saline and vaginal discharge on a microscope slide, add a coverslip, and examine for the actively motile parasite.

Microscopic preparations

Recommended tests
Gram-stained smears
KOH wet mount (fungi)
Saline wet mount (*Trichomonas*)

Skill level
Office trained
   Prepare Gram-stained smears
Medical technologist/technician
   Interpret Gram-stained smears and wet mounts

Equipment
Microscope

Reagent stability
No stability problems

Sources of error
Gram-stained smear with too much or too little color
Poorly collected and transported specimen
Misinterpreted microscopic results

Quality control
Check interpretation with experienced microbiologist
Compare interpretation with culture
Test reagents with stock organisms or known positive specimens

---

The potassium hydroxide (KOH) wet mount is useful for demonstrating yeast or fungi, as in cases of thrush or vaginitis caused by *Candida albicans*. Simply suspend a portion of the specimen in a drop of 10% KOH on a microscope slide, add coverslip, let stand for 15 to 30 minutes, and examine for yeast or fungal hyphae.

Skill level

Office or nursing personnel can prepare a Gram-stained smear or wet mount. A physician or trained medical technologist or technician should do the microscopic examination.

Equipment

A quality microscope with oil immersion lens is essential to interpret smears. Other items include a staining rack, microscope slides, coverslips, and immersion oil.

Gram-stain morphology of frequently encountered bacteria

Organism	Morphology	
A. Gram-positive cocci		
Streptococcus	Occur in short or long chains, occasionally in pairs	
Staphylococcus	Occur in irregular "grapelike" clusters; may appear singly, in pairs, short chains, or tetrads	
S. pneumoniae	Diplococcus, lancet-shape, oval; distal ends pointed; usually encapsulated.	
B. Gram-negative cocci or coccobacillus		
Neisseria	Diplococcus with adjacent sides flattened giving a "kidney bean" appearance; longer in width than length	
Acinetobacter Moraxella	Coccobacillus; may be pleomorphic; appear almost spherical; longer in length than width	
C. Gram-negative rods		
Enterics *E. coli Klebsiella*	Occur singly, in pairs, short chains; stain darker at ends; may be pleomorphic; barrel shape	
Pseudomonas	Occur singly, in pairs, short chains; rods are straight, more slender, less pleomorphic than enterics; stain evenly	
Haemophilus	Small coccobacillus; occur singly, in pairs, short chains; pleomorphic; stain faintly.	
D. Gram-positive rods		
Clostridium	Fat boxy rod with blunt ends; occur singly, in pairs; may be encapsulated	
Bacillus	Large rod; occur singly, pairs, short chains; ends may be rounded	
Corynebacterium (Diphtheroids)	Small rod; occur singly, pairs, short chains; pleomorphic; rounded or club-shaped ends; may occur in clumps	

Reagent stability

Commercial staining reagents are·stable for at least a year. The 10% KOH and saline should be replaced monthly, and reagents must not become contaminated with bacteria or fungi.

Sources of error

The major sources of error in microscopic examinations are poorly prepared smears and overinterpretation or misinterpretation of the results. The smear's technical adequacy must be assessed before trying to interpret it. If there is any doubt about its quality, a new smear should be made. Look in areas with PMNs to identify the pathogen; avoid areas showing many bacteria associated with SECs. Irregularly shaped gram-positive material with rough edges is most likely precipitated stain. Gram-positive organisms that are old or have been exposed to antibiotics or enzymes in body fluids or pus may appear gram negative. Last, faintly staining gram-negative bacilli such as *Haemophilus* species may be overlooked if the specimen contains protein material that stains pink. The best method for avoiding errors is to examine many specimens, compare your interpretation with culture results, and periodically confirm your results with a microbiologist.

Quality control

The Gram-stain reagents should be checked periodically— monthly, for example—with a Gram-positive and -negative organism, but the best QC is to assess the staining of routine specimens daily. All reagents should be periodically monitored for fungal contamination.

Expected accuracy

The accuracy of a microscopic examination in identifying an infectious agent depends on the expertise of the person examining the smear and the adequacy of the specimen. We will discuss the correlation of smear results with culture as we address each type of specimen.

URINE CULTURE

UTI is one of the most common infectious problems seen in an office practice, and its management requires accurate information about the numbers and types of bacteria involved. Quantitative urine culture has thus become a standard microbiological procedure for differentiating UTI from simple contamination of the urine during collection. Critical factors in the reliability of culture results are the careful collection and transport of the urine specimens.

Recommended tests

The recommended standard quantitative culture uses a calibrated loop to deliver a specific volume of urine (0.001 mL or 0.01 mL) to sheep blood agar and MacConkey or eosin methylene blue agars (Table 14-4). The method: Incubate the plates at 35 C for 24 hours, examine them for growth of gram-positive and gram-negative organisms, and then determine colony forming units (CFUs) per mL of urine by counting the colonies and multiplying by the appropriate dilution factor (1,000 or 100). You may then send positive cultures to a reference laboratory for identification and susceptibility testing. The alternative is to make a presumptive identification of *Escherichia coli*, *Pseudomonas aeruginosa*, *Staphylococcus aureus*, coagulase-negative staphylococci, and *Streptococcus* by using colonial morphology, the Gram stain, and such simple spot tests as oxidase, catalase, and indole.

Another culture method for screening urine cultures uses one of a variety of commercially available kits, which are usually made up of a paddle, slide, or tube coated with one or two media. The paddle or slide type is coated on each side with either a selective or nonselective medium; it is dipped into the urine, drained, and incubated in a sterile container. The CFU/mL is estimated by comparing the growth with standards in the kit. Such systems are easy to use. Their major disadvantages are not being able to identify mixed cultures easily and not having isolated colonies for subsequent tests.

Another method used to screen for bacteriuria is a reagent stick that detects nitrite and leukocyte esterase in urine specimens. The sensitivity, specificity, and predictive value of a negative test (positive is defined by culture results of greater than 100,000 CFU/mL) are 87%, 71%, and 97%. This method's usefulness as a screening tool is limited by its diagnostic sensitivity: It misses more than 10% of all culture-positive specimens. Several new instruments are being evaluated that can detect bacteria in urine specimens, but they are expensive and designed primarily for high-volume laboratories.

TABLE 14-4

Urine cultures

Recommended tests
Catalase test
Coagulase test
Dipstick culture
Oxidase test
Standard quantitative culture

Skill level
Office trained
   Gram-stain smears
   Inoculate cultures
   Read cultures for bacterial growth
Medical technologist/technician
   Interpret cultures and Gram-stained smears

Equipment
Bacteriologic loops (only for standard culture or identifying isolate)
Electric incinerator or alcohol lamp (only for standard culture or identifying isolate)
Incubator
Microscope
Refrigerator (only for plated media)

Reagent stability
Media are sensitive to dehydration and contamination
Test reagents are sensitive to heat and contamination

Sources of error
Corroded calibrated loop
Inappropriate incubation
Misinterpreted results
Outdated or contaminated media and test reagents
Poorly collected and stored specimen

Quality control
Test media and reagents with stock organisms
Monitor equipment temperature

A Gram stain of unspun urine is a useful method to detect an organism rapidly, presumptively identify it, and assess the quality of the specimen and subsequent culture results.

Skill level

Office or nursing personnel can inoculate culture media, prepare Gram-stained smears, and screen cultures for bacterial growth. A physician or trained technologist or technician should interpret culture results and do any biochemical tests.

Equipment

For the standard culture technique, the laboratory will need a refrigerator, incubator, electric incinerator or alcohol lamp, and disposable calibrated bacteriologic loops. For the commercial kits, only an incubator is necessary. The biochemical test reagents can be purchased from media supply houses.

Reagent stability

Commercial media are stable for three to six months from date of manufacture depending upon the media, storage conditions, and packaging. Media are susceptible to dehydration and contamination, and commercial products all have storage instructions and an expiration date on the package. The stability of the oxidase and coagulase reagent varies with the manufacturer. Hydrogen peroxide and the indole reagent are stable for one year.

Sources of error

Failure to collect, transport, or store a urine specimen properly often results in overgrowth of contaminating bacteria. Specimens should be refrigerated if they cannot be cultured within two hours after collection. Other problems include damaged or corroded calibrated loops, outdated or dehydrated media, and inappropriate incubation conditions. Patient-related problems include use of an antimicrobial agent, state of hydration, and frequency of urination.

Quality control

QC requirements discussed in the general culture procedure section apply here. In addition, the media and reagents for biochemical tests should be checked with known control organisms. Incubator and refrigerator temperatures should be monitored every day they are used. And when using the calibrated loop technique, it must be checked for damage every month or quarterly if used infrequently. This can most easily be done by contracting for the service with your reference laboratory. Coagulase reagent QC should be done as recommended by the manufacturer. Hydrogen peroxide, oxidase reagent, and the indole reagent should be checked for reactivity every two weeks.

Expected accuracy

Culture reliability of a single clean-catch specimen yielding greater than 100,000 CFU/mL is about 80% in women and nearly 100% in men. Two consecutive specimens from a woman approximates 95% accuracy. Stamm has recently demonstrated that symptomatic women often have urine coliform counts ranging from 100 to 100,000 CFU/mL and therefore may not be diagnosed by the standard urine culture. If more than 100 CFU/mL is considered significant in these patients, the urine culture has a sensitivity of 95%. A prudent approach to defining bacteriuria is to use 100,000 CFU/mL for asymptomatic women and 100 CFU/mL for symptomatic women.

GENITAL CULTURE

Genital tract infections are caused by bacteria, fungi, parasites, chlamydiae, and viruses, almost all of which are difficult to isolate and identify. The office microbiology laboratory should therefore culture primarily for *N. gonorrhoeae*, use a wet mount to diagnose vaginitis due to *Trichomonas* or *C. albicans*, and do a Gram-stained smear to diagnose nonspecific vaginitis. Cultures for other organisms should be sent to a reference laboratory.

Recommended tests

Specimens should be inoculated onto a standard selective medium such as modified Thayer-Martin agar and incubated in 5% CO_2 at 35 C for up to 72 hours. For the CO_2 atmosphere, use a candle jar, or a CO_2-generating tablet placed in a commercially available zip-lock bag or sealed chamber. For a fast, presumptive diagnosis of *N. gonorrhoeae*, prepare a Gram-stained smear on all genital specimens (Table 14-5). Presumptively identifying any growth on Thayer-Martin medium as *N. gonorrhoeae* requires a Gram smear (gram-negative diplococci) and an oxidase test (positive). The oxidase test can be performed directly on the colony or

Culture for *N. gonorrhoeae*

Recommended tests
Standard culture
Dipslide culture

Skill level
Office trained
   Gram-stain smears
   Inoculate cultures
   Read for bacterial growth
Medical technologist/technician
   Identify isolates
   Interpret cultures and Gram-stained smears

Equipment
Bacteriologic loops
Electric incinerator or alcohol lamp
Incubator
Microscope

Reagent stability
Media are susceptible to dehydration and contamination
Test reagents are susceptible to heat

Sources of error
Antibiotics in medium inhibiting *N. gonorrhoeae*
Improper incubation conditions
Outdated media and test reagents
Poorly collected and transported specimen

Quality control
Monitor incubation conditions
Test media and reagents with stock organisms

---

by smearing a portion of the colony on a filter paper with oxidase reagent. Confirming the isolate as *N. gonorrhoeae* should be done by a reference laboratory using biochemical or serologic tests.

Skill level

Office or nursing personnel can inoculate the media, prepare and stain smears, and read cultures for bacterial growth. A physician or trained technologist or technician should identify an isolate as *N. gonorrhoeae* and interpret the Gram smear.

Equipment

Culture techniques and presumptive identification of *N. gonorrhoeae* require a microscope, refrigerator, incubator, and electric incinerator or alcohol lamp. Commercial slide culture kits do not require sterile loops for inoculation.

Reagent stability

Isolating *N. gonorrhoeae* depends on the use of fresh media. To maintain quality, all media should be refrigerated, with careful attention to the manufacturer's expiration dates. Gram-stain reagents and commercial oxidase reagents are stable for six months to a year.

Sources of error

N. gonorrhoeae is a fastidious organism, susceptible to temperature changes and desiccation. Your laboratory may fail to isolate it by culture for a variety of reasons: inappropriate specimen collection or transportation (speculum lubricants, refrigeration, or dehydration, for example), outdated or dehydrated media, antibiotics in the medium that inhibit some strains (this has been known to cause a 3% to 10% false-negative rate), improper incubation, and misinterpretation of culture or test results.

Quality control

QC requirements discussed in the general culture section apply to genital cultures. It is most important to determine that the isolation system supports the growth of *N. gonorrhoeae* and inhibits other bacteria. The oxidase reagent should be checked for appropriate activity every two weeks with control organisms.

Expected accuracy

The Gram smear's sensitivity for diagnosing gonococcal infection in cervical material is about 55%, but specificity is high. A positive smear of urethral exudate from a male is nearly always diagnostic. The wet mount will detect trichomonads in 65% of the cases as compared to culture. Budding yeast and pseudohyphae will be found in the KOH preparation from most patients with significant vulvovaginal candidiasis.

A cervical culture for *N. gonorrhoeae* has a sensitivity of 80%, while a urethral culture from men has a sensitivity of nearly

100%. Anorectal cultures in women will detect another 10% to 15% of infections.

THROAT CULTURES

Pharyngitis is caused by a variety of organisms, most often viruses, and it is nearly impossible to determine the etiologic agent solely by clinical symptoms. Throat cultures identify *Streptococcus pyogenes* (group A beta-hemolytic streptococcus), the primary cause of bacterial pharyngitis in children and adults. In some specific situations, it may be necessary to culture for other organisms; these specimens should be sent to a reference laboratory.

Recommended tests

The standard culture for group A streptococcus involves vigorously swabbing the tonsillar and posterior pharyngeal area and plating the specimen on sheep blood agar (Table 14-6). After streaking the plate, a cut is made with the loop in the area of heaviest inoculum to enhance beta-hemolytic activity. Incubate the plate at 35 C, and read it at 24 and 48 hours. Test beta-hemolytic colonies for catalase to eliminate the possibility of hemolytic staphylococci and *Escherichia coli*. Since it is impossible to distinguish the growth of non-group A from group A beta-hemolytic streptococci, further tests are necessary to make the distinction. Some physicians feel that many beta-hemolytic streptococci in a symptomatic child are grounds for treatment since the isolate is probably group A. Otherwise, it can be presumptively identified by bacitracin susceptibility testing or specifically by serologic tests such as slide agglutination.

Another culture technique uses a commercial kit similar to urine dipstick methods. The blood agar, containing antibiotics to inhibit normal flora, is heavily inoculated with the throat swab and incubated at 35 C for 24 hours. Any beta-hemolytic colonies are presumed to be group A.

Several commercial slide agglutination systems detect group A streptococcus antigen extracted from throat swabs. The test can be completed within 10 to 85 minutes, depending upon the manufacturer, and requires little technical expertise. The sensitivity and specificity of these systems are about 90% and 97%, respectively. Based on material and personnel costs, these tests

Throat cultures

Recommended tests
Bacitracin susceptibility test
Catalase test
Dipstick culture
Serologic test for streptococci
Standard culture

Skill level
Office trained
    Inoculate and read cultures for beta-hemolytic streptococci
Medical technologist/technician
    Identify isolates
    Interpret cultures

Equipment
Bacteriologic loop (standard culture method)
Electric incinerator or alcohol lamp (standard culture method)
Incubator
Refrigerator (standard culture method)

Reagent stability
Media are susceptible to dehydration and contamination
Test reagents are susceptible to heat

Sources of error
Improper incubation conditions
Misinterpreted culture and test results.
Poorly collected and transported specimen
Outdated media and test reagents

Quality control
Monitor equipment temperature
Test media and reagents with stock organisms

are more expensive than a routine culture, but can often be done while the patient waits.

Skill level

Office or nursing personnel can easily learn the techniques needed to inoculate media and determine the presence or absence of beta-hemolytic streptococci. A physician or trained technologist or technician should interpret culture results and identify the organism by biochemical testing.

Equipment needed

When using the standard culture technique, the laboratory will need a refrigerator, incubator, and electric incinerator or alcohol lamp. Commercial slide cultures require only an incubator and refrigerator. Identifying beta streptococci by slide agglutination may necessitate buying a rotator.

Reagent stability

Commercial media are stable for three to six months from the date of manufacture depending on the medium, packaging, and storage conditions. Media are especially susceptible to dehydration and contamination. Bacitracin disks must be refrigerated, but are stable for at least a year. The stability of slide agglutination kits varies from three months to a year, depending on the manufacturer.

Sources of error

Your laboratory may fail to isolate and identify group A streptococcus for several reasons: poorly collected or transported specimens; the patient's use of antimicrobial agents, antibacterial mouthwash, or throat lozenge; outdated or dehydrated media; improper incubation; or misinterpretation of culture and test results. False-positive results may occur in patients who have viral pharyngitis but are streptococcal carriers.

Quality control

QC requirements discussed in the general culture procedure section also apply here. Media and test reagents should be checked with appropriate stock organisms. Since the dipstick culture system contains antibiotics to inhibit staphylococci and gram-negative bacilli, it must be checked with these organisms. Bacitracin

Factors that contribute to erroneous results

Falsely low (negative) values	Falsely high (positive) values
Urine	
1. Ineffective, outdated, dehydrated media	1. Skin contamination
2. Rapid diuresis	2. Improper storage of sample with bacterial overgrowth
3. Patient receiving antibiotic therapy	
Genital culture—*N. gonorrhoeae*	
1. Using incorrect incubator temperature	1. Using inappropriate source for Gram-stain diagnosis (throat or cervix)
2. Poor specimen collection	2. Misinterpreting the culture or test results
3. Loss of CO_2 from the bottle, jar, or plastic pouch	
4. Patient receiving antibiotics	
5. Using speculum lubricants	
6. Using ineffective, outdated, or dehydrated media	
7. Refrigerating the specimen or letting it dehydrate	
8. Delaying the initial culturing of specimen	
9. Inhibition of some strains by antibiotics in the media	
10. Misinterpreting the culture or test results	
Throat	
1. Poor collection technique	1. Beta-hemolytic strep carrier with a viral infection
2. Incubator out of 35-37 C range	2. Overreading beta hemolysis
3. Failing to get plates to room temperature before streaking	3. Overreading A disk zone of inhibition
4. Not streaking swab immediately or regard to beta hemolysis	4. Reading A disk zone without putting it in preservative
5. Patient receiving antibiotics	5. Using wrong A disks
6. Ineffective, outdated or dehydrated media	6. Reading a plate after more than 24 hours of incubation
7. Failing to make stabs	
8. Using faulty or outdated A disks or placing A disk on primary plate	
9. Misinterpreting culture or test results	

disks should be checked every month with a known isolate of group A streptococcus. QC of commercial serologic kits should be done as the manufacturer recommends. The hydrogen peroxide used in the catalase test should be checked every two weeks with a known beta-hemolytic group A streptococcus.

Expected accuracy

The sensitivity of standard or commercial slide culture is about 90%. The bacitracin test is very sensitive (96% to 99.8%), but much less specific (85% to 95%). A serologic method is the best identification procedure.

Table 14-7 outlines common factors that can contribute to erroneous results.

GENERAL REFERENCES

Bannatyne RM, Clausen C, McCarthy LR: Cumitech 10—Laboratory diagnosis of upper respiratory tract infections. Coordinating ed., Duncan IBR, Washington DC, American Society for Microbiology, 1979.

Barry AL, Smith PB, Turck M: Cumitech 2—Laboratory diagnosis of urinary tract infections. Washington DC, American Society for Microbiology, 1975.

Blazevic DJ, Hall CT, Wilson ME: Cumitech 3—Practical quality control procedures for the clinical microbiology laboratory. Washington DC, American Society for Microbiology, 1976.

Eschenbach D, Pollock HM, Schachter J: Cumitech 17—Laboratory diagnosis of female genital tract infections. Washington DC, American Society for Microbiology, 1983.

Fischer PM, Addison LA, Curtis P, et al: *The Office Laboratory*. East Norwalk, Conn. Appleton-Century-Crofts, 1983.

Gardner P, Provine HT: *Manual of Acute Bacterial Infections*. Boston, Little, Brown, 1976.

Gulick P, Hall G, McHenry MC: Office microbiology. *Med Clin North Am* 1983;67:39-55.

Kellogg Jr DS, Holmes KK, Hill GA: Cumitech 4—Laboratory diagnosis of gonorrhea. Coordinating eds., Marcus S, and Sherris JC, Washington DC, American Society for Microbiology, 1976.

Lennette EH, Balows A, Hausler WJ Jr, et al (eds): *Manual of Clinical Microbiology*, ed 4. Washington DC, American Society for Microbiology, 1985.

Stamm WE: Interpretation of urine cultures. *Clin Microbiol Newsletter* 1983;5:15-17.

15

Urinalysis, pregnancy, and infectious mononucleosis tests

CHEMICAL AND MICROSCOPIC URINALYSIS

In the hospital laboratory, a routine urinalysis consists of many tests including a chemical analysis, specific gravity measurement, and microscopic examination. Of these, some are more important in the ambulatory-care setting than others. It is important to be able to detect increased amounts of glucose or protein, microhematuria, and infection as indicated by the presence of bacteria or leukocytes, for example. Less important are the specific gravity, pH, and bilirubin.

With the reagent sticks now available from several manufacturers, you can confidently detect significant bacterial infection, microhematuria, glucosuria, and proteinuria in the ambulatory-care setting. A list of urinalysis test systems can be found in Appendix 1.

Recommended tests

Fresh urine, preferably a first morning specimen, should be tested no more than two hours after voiding with a strip capable of detecting glucose, protein, RBCs and hemoglobin, nitrite, and leukocyte esterase (Table 15-1). If the nitrite, leukocyte esterase, or protein tests are positive, the urine should be examined micro-

Urine tests

Recommended tests
  Dipstick tests
    Glucose
    Hemoglobin and RBC
    Nitrite
    Protein
    WBC leukocyte esterase

Skill level
  Office trained for dipstick
  Two-year medical lab technician for microscopic examination

Equipment needed
  Adequate light
  Adequate timer
  Centrifuge for microscopic examination
  Refractometer for specific gravity

Reagent stability
  Dipsticks are sensitive to moisture and heat

Sources of error
  Contamination
  Inadequate light
  Spoiled reagents
  Timing errors

Quality control
  Test artificial urine sample daily
  Compare every microscopic examination with dipstick results

scopically and cultured because urinary tract infection (UTI) is highly probable. A microscopic examination should also be done if red cell or hemoglobin tests are positive.

Skill level required

A person with minimal training can perform urine test strip procedures. Anyone who does these procedures, however, should first read the package insert and perform tests on several samples and control material closely supervised by someone with experience. Manufacturers' representatives will frequently provide training for new office personnel. This is a valuable service that you should use to advantage.

Microscopic examination of urine requires considerable training and experience. It should be undertaken only by a person with some level of formal laboratory training.

Equipment

Urine should always be collected in clean, well-rinsed containers because many chemical urinalyses give false results if the container is contaminated with cleaning materials. A clock with a second hand or a stopwatch is also necessary for accurately timing urine dipstick reactions, which must be evaluated in good light. Natural-color, fluorescent lighting is the best for accurate color comparison.

A centrifuge and a microscope with good 40× high dry objective are necessary for microscopic examinations. The microscope should have a built-in light source and a focusable condenser. Microscopic examinations are easier to evaluate if the sediment is stained; several manufacturers sell kits for preparing the stains.

Specific gravity can be measured several ways. The oldest method uses a urinometer, a modification of a hydrometer that floats in the urine; we do not recommend using it because of serious problems with miscalibrations. Most hospital and independent laboratories use a refractometer to measure specific gravity. This instrument is expensive but stable, and readings are not temperature sensitive. A specific gravity section has recently been added to some dipsticks, as well. Studies have shown that most readings are comparable within ±.005 units to refractometer readings when the pH is slightly acid, although high concentrations of glucose or x-ray contrast media can cause a greater discrepancy. The chemical dipstick reading correlates better with the urine osmolality than with the refractometer when these materials are present.

Reagent stability

Urine test strips deteriorate rapidly when exposed to heat or high humidity.

Sources of error

These are the major problems in urine testing:
- Testing a specimen that isn't fresh
- Collecting urine in a dirty or contaminated container
- Using deteriorated reagents
- Using improper testing technique
- Not mixing the urine specimen before testing
- Recording results incorrectly
- Failing to recognize or act on an abnormal result
- Misunderstanding interfering substances
- Making errors in timing
- Not having enough knowledge or experience to do the tests
- Evaluating the dipstick colors incorrectly because of poor lighting or color blindness

Several of these require special comment. The most common interfering substance in the urine of ambulatory patients is ascorbic acid.[1] About 50% of people tested for urinary ascorbic acid have concentrations that are detectable and could interfere with tests by inhibiting the enzymatic glucose reaction and the test for occult blood.[2]

A second significant source of error is the use of test strips with reagents that have deteriorated. Dipsticks are packaged with desiccating material because their reagent activity is degraded by moisture. They are also sensitive to excessive heat. The sticks must also be used before the expiration date marked on the container. The only reliable way to determine whether the test strips are functioning properly is to regularly use a quality-control sample with known concentrations of the test analytes. Another problem is failing to read results at the appropriate interval; they may be overestimated if they are read late and underestimated if they are read early. The package insert and the reference color chart clearly show when to read each reagent block after applying the specimen. This becomes fairly complicated in a reagent strip with nine different test blocks.

Technique in using the strip is important. It must never be dipped into urine and left there because the strip reagents will dissolve, diminishing the chemical reaction. After the strip is removed from the urine, it should be drained briefly against the side of the container and then placed horizontally so that the urine and chemicals from one block will not flow and contaminate the adjacent one.

As we mentioned, the microscopic examination of urine requires someone with laboratory training and experience, or misidentification of cells and other sediment is likely. A number of simple urine sediment examination systems using stains have been developed in the last few years.

Table 15-2 outlines common factors that can contribute to erroneous results.

Quality control

Regular quality-control (QC) procedures should be part of every laboratory test, whether done in the doctor's office or in a hospital or commercial laboratory. The results of QC testing should be recorded and the records kept for at least two years. QC testing is the physician's assurance that patient-care decisions are based on reliable testing information.

Urine dipsticks should be tested daily in a control solution containing all of the dipstick's constituents. These materials are commercially available in lyophilized, tablet, liquid, or dipstick form from a number of manufacturers (Ames, EM Science, General Diagnostics, and ICL Scientific). Dipsticks should be tested every day testing is done. People doing these tests should be checked for color blindness.

An experienced person should train each new employee in how to perform the test, interpret it, and use QC materials correctly. Whenever a microscopic examination of urine is performed, the results should be compared with the results of the urine dipstick. If there is a discrepancy, it should be investigated and resolved before reporting the results. If your laboratory does specific gravities, the refractometer should be checked daily with water and with control material to assure proper calibration.

Expected accuracy

In the College of American Pathologists (CAP) Proficiency Surveys,[3] about 99% of laboratories reported the correct answers for constituents tested by dipsticks. In a recent survey of doctor's office laboratories, 96% of the laboratories tested reported correct results. There are no data for the expected level of accuracy for

Factors that contribute to erroneous urinalysis results

Falsely low (negative) values	Falsely high (positive) values
Glucose (dipstick with glucose oxidase methodology)	
1. Ascorbic acid	1. Pyridium
2. Ketones (moderate concentrations)	
3. Salicylates (more than 2 g/day)	
4. Pyridium	
5. Deteriorated reagents in dipstick	
Glucose (reducing substances)	
	Ascorbic acid, cephalosporins, chloramphenicol, levodopa, metaxalone, methyldopa, nalidixic acid, penicillin (in high doses), salicylates (in high doses), streptomycin, sulfonamides, tetracycline, tyrosine
Ketones	
1. Aspirin	1. Highly pigmented urines
	2. High concentration of phenyl ketones
	3. Chlorpromazine, levodopa and phthalein compounds

microscopic urine examinations, but CAP Proficiency Surveys found that 87% to 97% of laboratories reported correct results in evaluating transparencies of urine sediment.

The office laboratorian should be aware of some of the limitations of commonly used urine reagent strips. One is their lack of reactivity with Bence-Jones (light-chain) proteins and fructose, which may be in the urine of pediatric patients with hereditary fructosuria. If there's a possibility of light-chain proteinuria, other methods must be used for detection and quantitation, and the urine of pediatric patients should be routinely screened for nonglucose reducing substances with other available methods such as Clinitest tablets from Ames.

Falsely low (negative) values	Falsely high (positive) values
Protein	
1. Dilute urine with dipstick	1. Strongly alkaline urine with dipstick
2. Highly alkaline urine with sulfasal method	2. Contamination with quarternary ammonium compounds with dipstick
	3. Tolbutamide, x-ray contrast media, penicillin, nafcillin, oxicillan, sulfasoxazole or turbid urine with sulfasal method
Blood	
1. High urine specific gravity or high protein concentrations	1. Microbial peroxidase in some urinary tract infections
2. Ascorbic acid	2. Bleach
Bilirubin	
1. Ascorbic acid (vitamin C) with dipstick	1. Ethoxazene, pyridium, phenothiazines, chlorpromazine
2. Pyridium and serenium with ictotest	2. Chlorpromazine (large amounts) with ictotest

PREGNANCY TESTING

Human chorionic gonadotropin (hCG) is a glycoprotein hormone consisting of two distinct amino acid chain subunits designated alpha and beta. It belongs to a family of pituitary and placental glycoprotein hormones, all of which contain closely related alpha subunits. They include follicle-stimulating hormone (FSH), luteinizing hormone (LH), and thyroid-stimulating hormone (TSH). The beta chain of each of these hormones differs, however, and is thought to confer biologic and immunologic specificity. The similarity of the alpha subunits, especially between hCG and LH, can cause problems in designing assays that measure only hCG with no interference from LH.

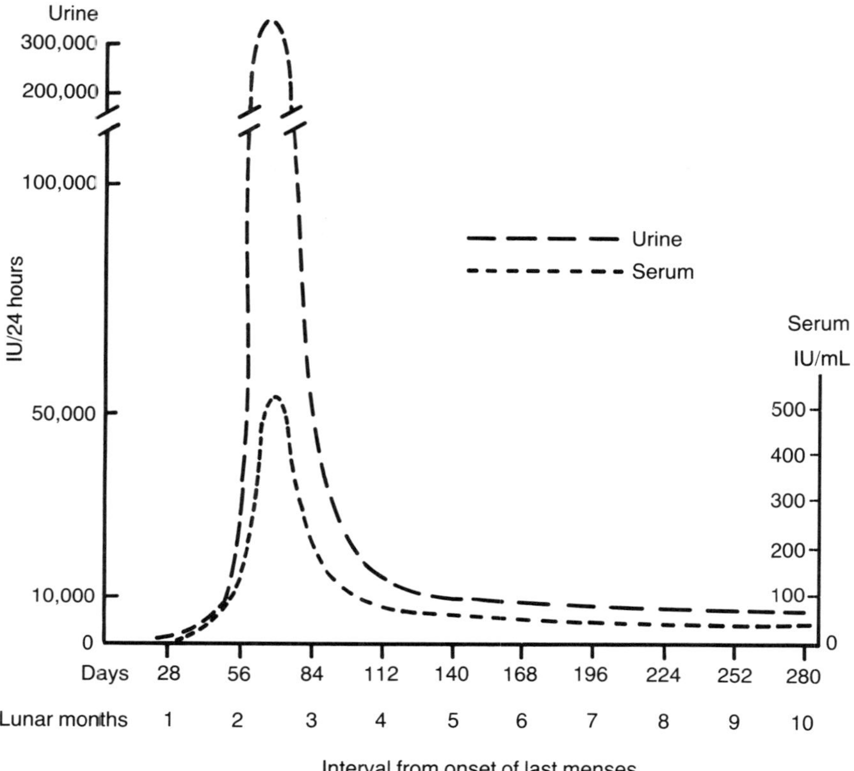

Source: Gold JJ, *Textbook of Gynecologic Endocrinology*, New York, Haber, 1968.

Trophoblastic cells of the placenta produce hCG. Its function is not fully defined, but it probably acts to maintain the corpus luteum after LH secretion decreases. The corpus luteum, in turn, produces progesterone and estrogens necessary for the survival of the pregnancy. Implantation of the fertilized ovum occurs about six to seven days after fertilization, and that's when hCG appears in maternal serum and urine, although not all assays can detect these low early levels.

In a normal pregnancy, hCG levels in maternal serum double about every two days, reaching a maximum level of 50,000 to 100,000 mIU/mL at 10 weeks' gestation (Figure 15-1). By 12 to

14 weeks, levels decline and remain at 10,000 to 20,000 mIU/mL. In an ectopic pregnancy, serum hCG levels increase more slowly than normal and usually remain below 6,000 mIU/mL. Serial hCG measurements along with ultrasound and physical diagnostic techniques can therefore be used to confirm or rule out an ectopic pregnancy. Levels of hCG are also increased in trophoblastic disease, usually much higher than in a normal pregnancy.

Pregnancy testing then is synonymous with testing for hCG. In this section we will review the common methods of assaying for hCG, note some of the pitfalls, and make some recommendations. A list of pregnancy tests can be found in Appendix 1.

Standardization

Until recently, all hCG assays were calibrated to the World Health Organization (WHO) Second International Standard for hCG (Second IS). This material was produced in 1963, and bioassay determined the International Unit. In about 1974, the WHO Biological Expert Committee prepared a new International Reference Preparation for hCG (First IRP) and redefined the International Unit. The First IRP is purer than the Second IS in that it contains a smaller amount of free alpha and beta chains. Since 1981, several reagent manufacturers have calibrated their assays to the new standard, which results in large discrepancies in results from assay to assay. For this reason, results from two different labs or even two different assays within the same lab should not be compared unless the calibration material or the correlation is known.

Specificity

In essence, all of today's tests are immunologic, involving antigen/antibody reactions to detect and quantify hCG. Because of the structural similarity between the gonadotropins and TSH and hCG, early pregnancy tests suffered from problems with cross-reactivity—the antibodies used could not completely distinguish between these hormones. Antibodies specific for the beta subunit of hCG have alleviated most of the cross-reactivity problems. As we mentioned, these assays give very different results depending on which standard is used for calibration. In the last few years, test kits using monoclonal antibodies against the beta and alpha subunits have been developed, and they have even greater specificity.

Slide tests for urinary hCG

These are still the most commonly used tests—so-called because they are done on a dark glass slide. They take one to three minutes to perform, detect hCG levels in the range of 500 to 4,000 mIU/mL, and are positive 10 to 14 days after the missed menstrual period.

There are many possible sources of error in this type of test. The technologist can unwittingly make the test positive or negative by agitating too much or too little, by not thoroughly mixing the reagents, or by misreading a small amount of agglutination as a positive test. Careful timing and temperature control are also crucial for consistent results, and any drying of the slide can cause false agglutination reactions; blood, protein, and some drugs can also cause false results. Now that more sensitive, simple-to-perform tests are available, no laboratory or physician should have to rely on this type of pregnancy testing.

Tube test for urinary hCG

The oldest and still the most commonly used tube tests use hemagglutination inhibition (HAI) to detect hCG. Sheep erythrocytes coated with hCG are mixed with anti-hCG antibody and the urine specimen. If the urine contains hCG, it will bind to the hCG antibody, the sheep red cells will not bind, and they will settle to the bottom of the tube in a characteristic ring formation—a positive result. If the urine contains no HCG, the added hCG antibody will make the red cells agglutinate, and they will form a smooth mat on the bottom of the tube—a negative result. The incubation time is usually in the one-to-two hour range, hCG can be detected down to a level of about 150 to 200 mIU/mL, and results are positive at about five to nine days after the missed menstrual period.

These tests have many possible sources of error. The tubes are inserted upright in a rack with a tilted mirror to let the technologist see the ring. During incubation, the rack must remain level and completely still, any bumping or vibration can cause a false reaction. The test is also very sensitive to temperature variations, and reaction must be read at the proper time to avoid false positives or negatives. Blood, protein, and some drugs may cause false reactions, and cloudy specimens should be filtered. In specimens with a specific gravity lower than about 1.012, the hCG level might be below the detectable limit; for this reason, many procedures require that a first morning specimen be used.

Another version of the tube test involves latex particles similar to the slide tests, but the reaction takes place and flocculation is read in a test tube. This test's characteristics are similar to the other tube tests. In general, these tests have fairly good sensitivity and if properly done can produce reliable results. Although they are more reliable than slide tests, we now have better alternatives.

Enzyme immunoassays for urinary hCG

A new generation of pregnancy tests has now become available that uses enzyme-labeled monoclonal antibodies. In these tests, a monoclonal antibody to the alpha subunit of hCG is coated on a plastic bead or on the inside of a plastic test tube. Urine is added, along with a second antibody directed against the beta subunit. These reactants incubate for 30 to 60 minutes, then the bead or tube is washed, and a substrate solution that will react with the enzyme attached to the second antibody is added. After this incubation, the amount of color in the tube is read by comparison with a known reference tube.

These are called sandwich assays, because hCG in the specimen is sandwiched between the two monoclonal antibodies. This type of assay can detect hCG down to 25 to 50 mIU/mL and can be positive seven to 10 days after conception, several days before the missed menstrual period. It detects only intact hCG, which is the main form of the hormone present in pregnancy. Since a wash step is included, interference from protein, blood, or drugs is virtually eliminated if the washing is done carefully. No ring or agglutination reaction is going on, so rocking or bumping the tubes will not cause errors. These assays' good sensitivity and ease of handling make them amenable to almost any laboratory situation.

Serum assays

We have had very sensitive assays for hCG for several years. The most common methods are radioimmunoassay (RIA) or enzyme immunoassay (EIA), and the procedures are designed to measure hCG down to about 2 mIU/mL. Such high sensitivity is not necessary for routine pregnancy testing but is sometimes needed to detect ectopic pregnancy or tumors. Most of these assays call

Pregnancy tests

Assay	Sensitivity	Time	Sources of error
Slide test	500-4000 mIU/mL	1-3 min	Temperature, too vigorous rocking, drying of plate, mixing, protein, blood, drugs, reading agglutination, dilute urine
Hemagglutination inhibition tube test	150-200 mIU/mL	1-2 hr	Temperature, bumping rack, protein, blood, drugs, dilute urine
Latex flocculation tube test	150-200 mIU/mL	1-2 hr	Temperature, protein, blood, drugs, dilute urine
Monoclonal antibody enzyme tube test	25-50 mIU/mL	1-2 hr	Inadequately washing bead or tube antibody

for radioactive materials that would not be manageable in a smaller laboratory.

A monoclonal sandwich-type assay using enzyme labeling is also available, which works and handles like the enzyme-labeled monoclonal antibody urine assay. But it requires a spectrophotometer and more complex data manipulation to get a quantitative result.

Recommended tests

To some extent, the setting in which the test will be used determines the method of choice. In most practices, the test is done to detect normal pregnancy, and we recommend a urine test using a monoclonal antibody enzyme immunoassay. The extreme sensitivity of 50 mIU/mL will detect some early pregnancies that will be carried only for a short time. For this reason, we recommend that results in the 50 to 200 mIU/mL range be reported as doubtful or borderline, and that a new urine sample be tested several days later (Figure 15-1 and Table 15-3).

Skill level required

Personnel with minimal training can process monoclonal antibody enzyme immunoassays if they carefully follow instructions supplied with the kit. Slide tests require greater technical skill and attention to technique.

Equipment

No special equipment is required for the recommended tests.

Reagent stability

Pregnancy test reagents have a finite life. Most kits require refrigeration and have an expiration date marked on the box and the reagent bottles.

Sources of error

Each new generation of pregnancy tests is less subject to error than the preceding one. In spite of this, occasional false-positive results are still reported for monoclonal antibody enzyme immunoassays. These methods' extreme sensitivity can lead to a positive report in some early pregnancies (if 50 mIU/mL is used to define positive) that will spontaneously abort within the next few days. Consequently, preference should be given to test kits that use 200 mIU/mL to define a positive result. False-negative results can occur because the concentration of hCG is below the detection limit either because it is very early in the pregnancy or because the urine is dilute. Reagent storage conditions are critical to proper functioning of these tests, and the kits must be used before the expiration date printed on the box and reagent bottles. Table 15-4 outlines common factors that can contribute to erroneous results.

Quality control

A positive control sample should be processed every day the test is performed. As we discussed, the strongly positive control supplied by the manufacturer should be diluted to yield a weakly positive sample that will mean a reduced sensitivity in detecting hCG.

Expected accuracy

Using the monoclonal antibody enzyme immunoassay with a positive defined as having more than 200 mIU/mL of urinary hCG, the false-positive rate (for normal pregnancy) is close to zero. Some manufacturers, however, have supplied only a 50 mIU/mL or a 100 mIU/mL standard, so these tests would have a measur-

Factors that contribute to erroneous pregnancy test results

Falsely low (negative) values	Falsely high (positive) values
Pregnancy test—urine	
1. Dilute urine	1. Proteinuria (with some latex agglutination tests)
2. Early pregnancy (before hCG secretion is detectable)	2. Using outdated or improperly stored reagents
3. Ectopic pregnancy (hCG levels low for dates)	3. hCG secreting tumors
4. Missed abortion	4. Inadequate mixing
5. Later pregnancy (when hCG levels are down) or when hCG levels are very high (prozone effect with some latex and hemagglutination techniques)	

able false-positive rate based on their redefinition of positive. The actual rate would depend on the number of women who are tested between the day of the expected menses and 10 to 14 days after the date of the missed period (as many as a third to a half of concepti may abort spontaneously during this interval). False-negative results can occur if the concentration of urinary hCG is below the positive standard because the urine is dilute or because the hCG secretion is below detectable levels—due to an abnormal implantation or a very early pregnancy.

Other urine tests may have specific technique-associated sources of error. Most slide tests, for example, are critically susceptible to forcing a false positive or a false negative by how the reagents are mixed. Hemagglutination techniques are subject to problems because minimally trained individuals have difficulty reading the end point. It also has problems with high protein in the specimen and with a prozone effect that gives false-negative results from extremely high concentrations of urinary hCG.

INFECTIOUS MONONUCLEOSIS

Usually a self-limited infection with Epstein-Barr virus (EBV), infectious mononucleosis (IM) can present diagnostic problems because of its varied manifestations. The disease, most common in adolescents and young adults, is usually marked by a vague onset that is not much different from that of other infections. One major reason to test for IM is to differentiate it from group A beta-hemolytic streptococcal infection, because the two illnesses can be otherwise indistinguishable. When patients have a prolonged relapsing disease course, vague systemic symptoms including fevers and prominent lymphadenopathy must be differentiated from other, more serious infection.

Since it is not practical to test for the virus itself, serologic tests for heterophil antibodies are used instead. A number of other conditions can cause heterophil antibodies in the blood, however. Since these immunoglobulins also agglutinate sheep red blood cells, most test systems include some way to increase assay specificity by minimizing the influence of all but those associated with IM.

Recommended tests

Kits are available to test for the presence of heterophil antibody in serum (Mono-Tek from ICL Scientific, Monosticon Dri-Dot from Organon Diagnostics, Mono-Test from Ortho Diagnostics, and Mono-Test from Wampole Laboratories) or in a whole blood specimen (Mono-Test-FTB from Wampole Laboratories).

Skill level required

Personnel with no formal laboratory training can do heterophil testing with these kits, but they will have to develop some skill in performing the test and in distinguishing a positive from a negative result. Some kits use simple, one-step methods; others require more complex testing that involves adsorption of heterophil antibodies that are not associated with IM. In general, it is wise to choose a relatively simple system if the staff has minimal or no formal laboratory training.

Equipment

These kits come complete with all reagents and other necessary materials.

Reagent stability

Reagents in kits that use fixed red cells are intrinsically more stable than those that use stabilized red cells. The latter are usable for up to six months if they are stored at refrigerator temperature (4 C) while the former are stable for 12 to 18 months under the same conditions. As we have stressed throughout, reagents should never be used for patient testing beyond the manufacturers' printed expiration date.

Sources of error

Since testing for heterophil antibody is not specific for IM, it should be used in association with evaluating a peripheral blood smear. The heterophil test can have very high sensitivity and specificity, but since it is most often used for screening in a low prevalence group, the predictive value of a positive result usually runs about 75% to 85%. Because it is frequently used to evaluate difficult diagnostic situations, it can be helpful but is usually not conclusive by itself.

False-negative results can occur in patients with IM if the test is performed too early in the clinical course. Repeat testing usually remedies this problem. Because of persistence of the heterophil antibody, false-positive results can occur in asymptomatic patients who have had the disease. False-positive results may also be associated with a number of conditions unrelated to IM, including viral hepatitis, rheumatoid arthritis, malaria, Hodgkin's disease, leukemia, and a few other malignant disorders.

Quality control

When a new reagent kit first comes into the office, it is important to ascertain that the reagents and the new controls are comparable to those currently being used. It is thus prudent to use both sets of reagents to test a single patient specimen.

Most heterophil reagent testing kits come with positive and negative controls, which are actually standards to help the user differentiate between both kinds of reaction. When using this material as a control, it is important to know the positive control's titer in order to evaluate whether it would be sensitive to minimal changes in the test conditions and reagent reactivity, and thus give early warning of problems with the method. True controls should be used at least once a day to ensure that the test system is operating appropriately; the results should be recorded in a log.

Some systems do not provide controls, but reading reference materials instead. With these systems, it may be appropriate to test sera taken from patients known to have a positive heterophil or to use other, true control material each day.

Expected accuracy

Both the sensitivity and specificity of the heterophil antibody detection test have been estimated to be as high as 98% to 99%, but the accuracy is a function of prevalence in the test population. If 20% of those tested can be expected to have mononucleosis, the predictive value of a positive result will be 96% (96 of 100 individuals with a positive test will really have the disease). If only 1% of the people tested can be expected to have mononucleosis, the predictive value of a positive result falls to 50% (only half of those with a positive test will actually have the disease).

REFERENCES

General references—Urinalysis

Young DS: Effect of Vitamin C on laboratory tests. *Lab Med* 1983;14:278-282.

Free AH, Free HM: Rapid convenience urine tests: Their use and misuse. *Lab Med* 1978;9:9-17.

Elevitch FR, Noce PS: Data Recap 1970-1980. Skokie, Ill., College of American Pathologists, 1981.

General references—Pregnancy testing

Fuchs F, Klopper A (eds): *Endocrinology of Pregnancy*, ed 2. Hagerstown, Md., Lippincott, 1977.

Speroff L, Glass RH, Kase NG: *Clinical Gynecologic Endocrinology and Infertility*, ed 3. Baltimore, Williams & Wilkins, 1983.

Statland BE: Updating pregnancy and urine assays. *Diagnosis* 1985;7: Special issue, September 1985, pp 47-52.

Williams RH (ed): *Textbook of Endocrinology*. Philadelphia, WB Saunders, 1981.

General references—Infectious mononucleosis

Branch WT, Weinstein L: Diseases of the upper respiratory tract, in Branch WT (ed): *Office Practice of Medicine*. Philadelphia, WB Saunders, 1982.

Davey FC, Nelson DA: Leukocyte disorders, in Henry JB (ed): *Clinical Diagnosis and Management by Laboratory Methods*. Philadelphia, WB Saunders, 1984.

Fisher PM, Addison LA, Curtis P, et al: *The Office Laboratory*. East Norwalk, Conn., Appleton-Century-Crofts, 1983.

Ray CG, Hicks MJ, Minnich LL: Viruses, Rickettsia, and Chlamydia, in Henry JB (ed): *Clinical Diagnosis and Management by Laboratory Methods*. Philadelphia, WB Saunders, 1984.

16

Supervising patients' self-testing

Home testing is here to stay. Some of these procedures are already well established in our medical culture. One such area is home glucose monitoring; diabetic patients are quite accustomed to testing their urine and, more recently, blood to estimate diabetic control. Among the newer tests sold for self-testing are pregnancy tests, tests for urine luteinizing hormone (LH) for estimating the time of ovulation, and various methods to detect occult blood in the stool.

Just as technology has dispersed to the office laboratory, many people are now using these home tests, and many more will soon be available—in spite of the skepticism on the part of professional laboratorians. We will discuss quality assurance in the office laboratory in the next chapter. The issues and the instruments in self-testing are very similar, but in this case, the physician must play the role of consultant and help the patient produce reliable results. We will use home glucose monitoring as an example of how to manage such a quality-assurance program for your patients who do self-testing.

BASIS OF THE LABORATORY DIAGNOSIS

Reagent stick methods for determining blood glucose are usually performed with capillary blood but may also be done with venous blood. Appropriate reference values must be used in each case, of course; they are usually different. The procedure is simple: The blood is put directly on the reagent pad that is covered by a semipermeable membrane through which glucose can diffuse but red cells cannot. After an appropriate length of time, the blood is wiped or washed from the surface of the pad, and the value is determined with a reflectance meter or by comparison with a set of printed standards. Although the reagents are completely prepackaged and the equipment is called self-checking and adjusting, some variance in the testing process is expected and, in untrained hands, can be significant (Chapter 17).

SOURCES OF ERROR

A number of factors before and during the testing process can cause errors. Irregular timing of specimen collection in relation to meals and snacks is a constant problem with blood glucose testing. Test timing should be regularized so the results from any one day can confidently be compared with those of other days. When the patient is using home monitoring, changes in the insulin dosage schedule should not be based on a single result but rather on changes in the glucose control pattern using a number of data points.

Changes in reagent reactivity can also cause errors. Expiration dates on reagent containers should be rigorously adhered to. In addition, the strips are quite vulnerable to moisture, so it's important to keep the package tightly closed and to be sure the moisture-absorbant pack in the package is in place.

Testing errors can also occur during the analysis: a timing error, putting more or less blood on the strip, or variability in cleaning the blood from the strip. The reading can also be distorted because of poorly calibrated reflectance meters or because the patient wants to report a better value or has problems with visual acuity.

QUALITY CONTROL

The results of home glucose monitoring are, potentially, translated directly into a management decision—the insulin dosage schedule—without consulting the physician. Consequently, reducing the potential for error to a minimum is essential to patient safety. One way is to use capillary glucose monitoring as a means of determining when the patient should consult the physician about changing the insulin dosage. This will let the physician determine whether the changes are necessary or there are other problems that require medical attention.

Ordinarily, patients simply take responsibility for adjusting insulin dosage between office visits. Under these circumstances, they must be taught about the testing process and strongly encouraged to keep complete records. Monitoring four times a day would be ideal, but not at all practical; patients should therefore arrange their testing so that several values each week are from each of the testing times; before breakfast, mid-morning or before lunch, before dinner, and before bedtime. It is also most important that patients using reflectance meters scrupulously observe the manufacturer's recommendations regarding calibration, maintenance, cleaning, and control procedures. All patients should periodically test control samples to make sure that the system is functioning properly and producing expected results. These control sera results should be recorded in the log just as their own blood glucose results are.

The physician should have a program for teaching patients the correct way to do the analysis (perhaps including audiovisual materials that allow some self-paced learning). The doctor should also have a way to test mastery of the technique (including predetermined standards that call for further education) and to make sure that the patient does not have a physical problem, such as poor vision or color blindness, that would preclude reliable results. A record should be kept of the teaching session, and the self-test results noted in the patient's medical record.

When the patient is seen in the office, a capillary glucose determination should be compared with a laboratory-performed analysis on a specimen collected at the same time. If the discrepancy between the two exceeds some predetermined limit (15% is reasonable) or the results in the self-testing log are discordant with those found in the office, the clinician should try to find the source of the problem. As noted, this could result from a change in the patient's physical condition, such as a deterioration in visual acuity. If the problem is a result of poor technique, the physician's staff should undertake remedial training to improve the reliability of the patient's results.

GENERAL REFERENCE

1. Bradley M, Schumann GB: Examination of urine, in Henry JB (ed): *Clinical Diagnosis and Management by Laboratory Methods,* ed 17. Philadelphia, WB Saunders, 1983.

17

Quality assurance

This chapter presents an introduction to quality assurance as well as a list of key terms. We also discuss sources of variation in the analytic process, ways to minimize error, the importance of preventive equipment maintenance, how to validate the reliability of day-to-day results, how to approach results outside acceptable limits, and the importance of accurate reporting.

Practicing clinicians have been held responsible for interpreting laboratory data and for the resultant patient-management decisions—and until recently, they have relied on the professional laboratorian for accurate test information. But now that test analysis is returning to the office laboratory, practicing physicians will be responsible for the entire process: the accuracy of the laboratory information as well as that of the interpretation and management decisions.

Laboratorians have long been aware of the complexities of the testing process and have developed protocols to minimize the likelihood of errors affecting test results. Table 17-1 shows how vulnerable the testing process is to error. The details of potential errors are different in the office laboratory, but the physician must be able to validate that a result is accurate and precise and that it belongs to a particular patient.

Text continues on page 244

Potential sources of error determined in a hospital laboratory*

Action	Potential error

Test ordered after history taking and physical exam	Wrong test is ordered
	No history of conditions affecting test interpretation
	    Incomplete dietary history
	    Incomplete drug history
	    Incomplete evaluation of recent tests and procedures

Physician writes an order in the patient's chart	Handwriting is illegible
	Orders are written on the wrong form or the wrong place in the chart
	Test requirements are not specified
	    Fasting or random sample
	    Time of day
	    Test frequency
	    Relationship to other diagnostic procedures

Nurse or secretary transcribes the order to a requisition slip	Patient chart is not properly flagged Patient chart is in the wrong place or temporarily misplaced Orders are misread or charts with written orders are overlooked Information is transcribed to the wrong form Lab form is improperly filled out, unclear, or illegible Important details of the order are not transcribed The wrong patient's name is used on the lab requisition The laboratory requisition is not verified against the original order
Laboratory requisition is delivered to the laboratory	Requisition is misplaced on the ward Transportation delays or pickup was the time designated for the test Requisition is delivered to the wrong department or the wrong place in the lab Messenger loses the requisition

Action	Potential error

Requisition is received and logged into the laboratory	Requisition is misplaced or lost by the lab clerk
	    It sticks to another form, is thrown away, or put in the wrong file
	    The clerk is distracted and fails to complete the transcription
	Information is transcribed incorrectly
	    Patient name, hospital number, lab numbers, or names of tests

Blood pick-up slips are prepared and given to a phlebotomist	Wrong information is written on the slips
	    Wrong patient's name is on the slip
	    Test list is incomplete or illegible
	    First name (or middle initial) confusion in patients with same last (or first and last) name
	Slip never reaches the phlebotomist

Phlebotomist goes to the ward to draw blood from the patient	Phlebotomist draws wrong patient—does not correctly match slip with name on armband
	Phlebotomist uses the wrong tube
	    Incorrect anticoagulant causing interference with the test
	    Inadequate sample volume is collected
	Phlebotomist allows blood hemolysis causing interference with test
	Blood is drawn at wrong time or out of phase with initial order

Phlebotomist returns blood to the laboratory	Substance to be measured deteriorates because of a delay in returning to the lab, improper handling during transport, excessive agitation, or exposure to adverse environmental conditions (ie., failure to keep cool) Serum or plasma hemoconcentration is lost, or contamination occurs because of dropped tube or leakage of separated serum or plasma

continued

Action	Potential error
Specimen is logged in, work sheet prepared	Transcription errors
	Worklists do not contain complete list of tests to be processed
	Wrong patients or tests appear on wrong work lists
Specimen is processed: Centrifugation and transfer of plasma serum to other tubes	Centrifugation causes hemolysis due to heat or excess speed
	Tube breaks in centrifuge with potential for contamination of other specimens
	Specimens are transposed during centrifugation or serum separation
	Transfer tubes are dirty or contaminated
	Transfer tubes are mislabeled
	Transfer tubes are not matched to work lists
Specimens and worklists are taken to processing area	Technologist is not informed of tests to be done
	Worklist or specimen is lost or misplaced
	Technologist does the test on wrong tube or wrong test on right tube
	Series of tests are put in incorrect sequence
Analysis is performed	Reagent errors
	Mislabeled
	Out-dated
	Incorrectly formulated
	Contain precipitates or contamination
	Incorrect pipette is used or the pipette is incorrectly calibrated or read
	Read-out instrument is improperly calibrated
	Dirty cuvettes
	Wrong wavelength is selected
	Phototube is weak
	Incorrect zero or null-point calibration

Action	Potential error
	Calibration curves are incorrectly formulated or are not updated often enough
	Insufficient or no controls are included in the run
	Reagents are added to sample in different sequence than standards or controls
Reading, recording and calculation of results	Technologist misreads the instrument
	Reading is incorrectly transcribed to the worksheet or answer log
	Calculations are incorrect because of math errors, transposed decimal points, use of the wrong formula, or failure to include physical factors or mathematical constants in the final calculations
	Results are transcribed to the wrong column on worksheet or record or into another patient's file
Results are transcribed from worksheet to patient's record and placed in lab file for retrieval	Information is incorrectly transcribed
	Results are placed in the wrong column or listed against the wrong test
	Results are placed in the wrong patient's lab report
	Lab data are misfiled or in a form that makes retrieval impossible
	Results on the formal lab report do not match telephoned results
Lab reports are taken to the floor for charting	Messenger is delayed
	Pneumatic tube malfunctions
	Report is lost in transit or misplaced on the ward or chart is not in rack
	Report is placed in the wrong patient's chart or the wrong place in the chart

continued

Action	Potential error
Physician reads the report, assimilates data into making a diagnosis, or formulates a management decision	Physician fails to read the test result Data are not clearly presented Data are faintly copied, crowded, or unrecognized because of unfamiliar form or placement Important results are not adequately flagged Important data are lost in mass of normal values or not seen because of misplacement among other reports that are out-of-date sequence The physician does not remember ordering the test and does not anticipate the results Results are incorrectly correlated with previous results or other tests, and the physician interprets them incorrectly

* Adapted from an analysis made at General Rose Memorial Hospital, Denver.

ACCURACY AND PRECISION IN LABORATORY TESTING

Assessing a patient and developing a diagnostic or management strategy include the evaluation of laboratory data in the context of all other clinical findings. Reliable—or as the glossary defines it, accurate and precise—laboratory data are essential to the decision-making process. Years ago, each laboratory tried to control each procedure using its own locally developed standard solutions, biologically active preparations, and control materials derived from surplus patient sera. With these materials, it was difficult to maintain the consistency of results within a particular laboratory and virtually impossible to achieve uniform standards of accuracy between laboratories. This meant that a clinician often had to use a different point of reference for the same test on the same patient being tested in two or more different settings.

The development of large automated instruments brought about a major advance in laboratory medicine: procedures, protocols, and materials to ensure testing quality and to provide a basis for standardizing test results. This is the foundation of today's high-quality laboratory results that provide the information we need for diagnostic and management decisions.

As technology has continued to improve, it is now possible to return much of the testing process to the physician's office laboratory. But this testing must also be subject to rigorous quality control. Perhaps it is even more important in the office laboratory because people with minimal technical training will often perform the tests and because many of the test results are likely to be translated directly into patient management decisions. The practitioner must therefore understand testing principles and pitfalls and have working protocols that will ensure the validity of test results.

VARIATION IN THE TESTING PROCESS

Testing variation is defined by a statistical analysis of the results of processing a single specimen a number of times with the same machine, the same method, and the same reagents. Because of complexities in the testing process, any automated or manual chemistry procedure will produce not one but a group of results (Figure 17-1). Good test procedures will be very precise in the sense that all results will be close to the mean (Figure 17-2); in other words, the standard deviation, which defines the size of the spread, will be small.

Laboratorians use the term coefficient of variation (CV) to describe this variation in the testing process. The CV, which is a standard deviation of the set of results divided by the mean value, is convenient to use because it is independent of the numeric values of the mean and the units that produce it. We can use the CV to determine 95% confidence limits of any reported value. For example, the CV of a WBC count done in our hospital laboratory was found to be 2%, while the CV of the same procedure on a semiautomated cell counter in a physician's office laboratory was 8%. This means that the determined value of a count of 12,000 cells/μL from hospital cell counter would be within 11,520 to 12,480 ($\pm$ 2 standard deviations) 95% of the time, while the same range for the office counter would be 10,080 to

Normal statistical distribution curve

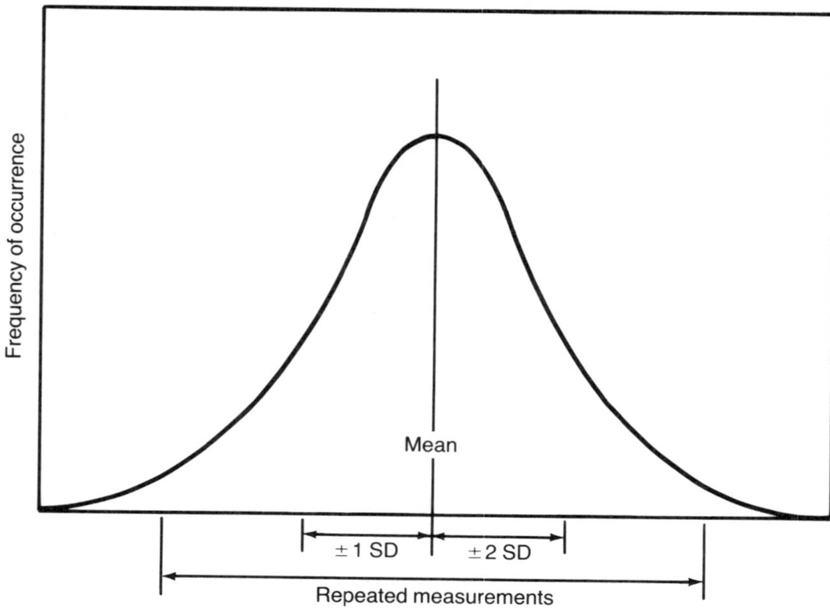

This Gaussian curve shows that ± 1 SD from the mean encompasses 68% of the data points, ± 2 SD includes 95% of the data points.

13,920 (Figure 17-3); 5% of the results would be even farther from the mean value because of variation in the testing process.

It is easy to see that the "true value" of the Coulter count is right at the upper limit of the value expected in a healthy population and the testing variation is small enough to let the physician interpret it reliably. The variation implicit in the alternate method is such that it would be hard to tell whether the result was clearly normal (10,000), borderline (12,000), or clearly abnormal (14,000). In this example, there is obviously a trade-off between speed and reliability of results.

QUALITY ASSURANCE IN LABORATORY TESTING

The variability in determining the white blood cell count can be attributed to the laboratory testing process itself, including variability in the equipment function, the reagents, and the individ-

Laboratory precision and accuracy defined

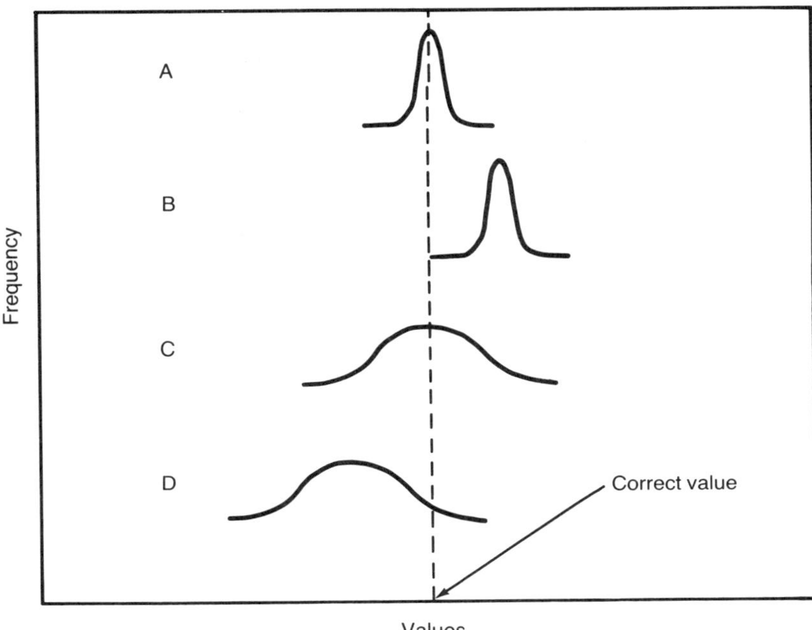

These are frequency distributions showing results of repeatedly testing a single control sample or patient specimen. Precise test results do not vary widely from their own mean value (A and B), compared with less precise methods (C and D). In accurate test results, the mean value closely approximates the true value (A and C), compared with less accurate methods (B and D). Method A is more precise and accurate than the other methods, so its results more reliably approximate the true value.

ual doing the test. Quality assurance protocols make it possible to identify systematic sources of error that can develop in the testing process, but it is difficult to identify random errors unless they are so discordant with the patient's condition that the result strains credibility.

It is also important to realize that a substantial fraction of anomalous laboratory results (about half) are not attributable to test-processing problems. They come from other aspects of the cycle, including collecting and handling specimens and reporting results, as Table 17-1 shows. Although a large number of essentially unrelated problems can develop, a recurrent theme that is quite relevant to physician's office testing is how many errors oc-

How different coefficients of variation affect the distribution of determined values

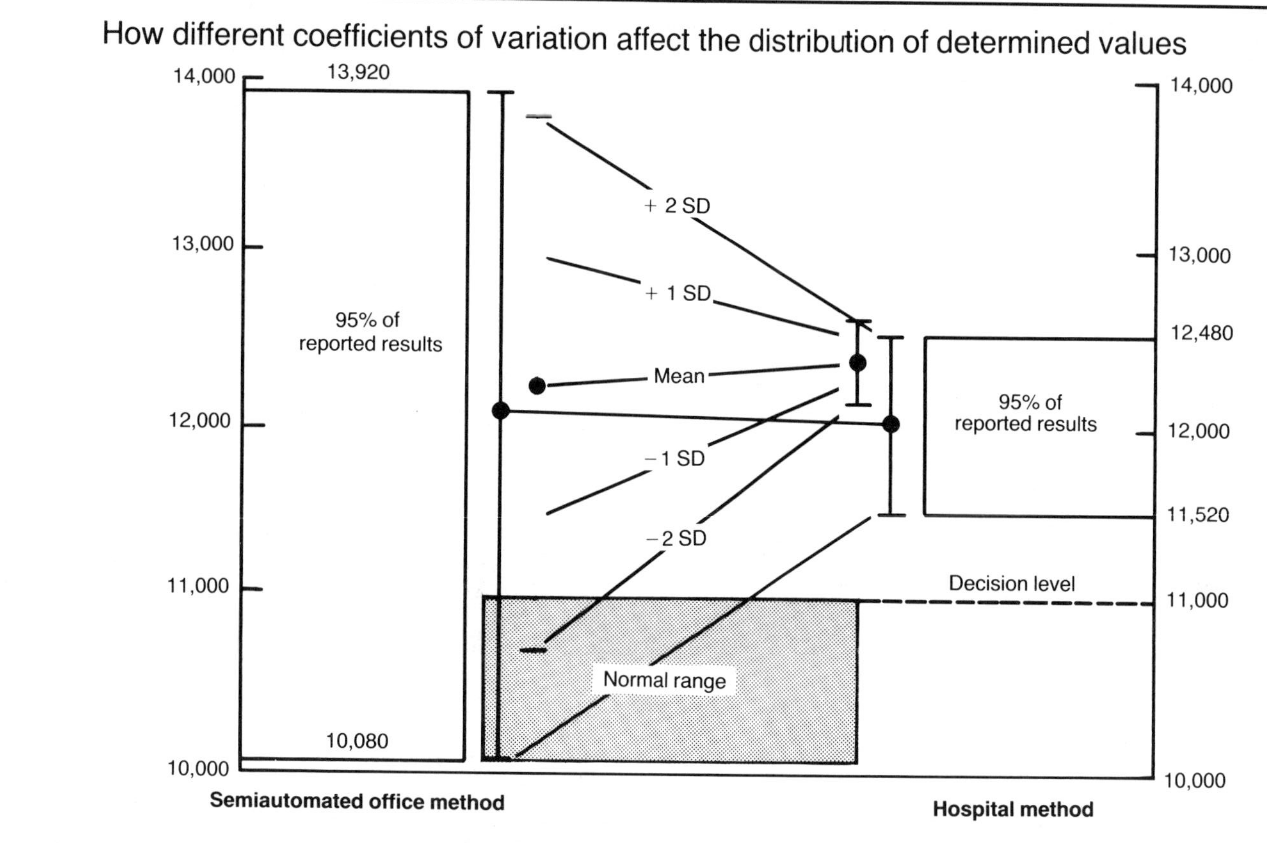

cur because of mistakes in such clerical functions as transcribing and filing.

When testing goes into the office practice, quality assurance protocols are essential. If any questions about a particular result should arise, the physician should be able to provide reasonable documentation that the result was accurate and precise and that the result was, in fact, relevant to the patient in question. Such a program must deal with problems that can develop before processing, with appropriate security measures after processing, and with variation in the testing process itself. It is important to note the patient's testing condition—fasting, hours after eating, or time of day, among others—for correct interpretation of the test result. We will discuss approaches to a broad-based quality assurance program later in this chapter and have already touched on specifics in chapters 12 through 16. In Chapter 7, we discuss the malpractice and liability implications of office testing and the role of quality assurance protocols in minimizing such risk.

CONCLUSIONS

To ensure the reliability of test information, the physician's office laboratory, like any other, must establish a quality assurance program. This gives the physician a firm basis for assuming responsibility for valid test results, for interpreting the results, and for making diagnostic and management decisions. Understanding the office laboratory technology is also basic to providing the quality test information that is essential for medical management decisions.

GLOSSARY

Accuracy: The extent to which measurements agree with the true value of the quantity being measured. It should not be confused with precision, which is how much results vary from each other.

Coefficient of variation: An index used to describe the precision of a laboratory method. It is calculated with this formula: CV = standard deviation ÷ mean.

Decision value: A threshold value above or below which a physician will respond with a particular action.

Precision: The reproducibility of a test result as described by its variation. The smaller the variation, the greater the precision.

Predictive value: The ability of a test to identify individuals with or without a particular problem (positive and negative, respectively) in a defined population using a defined threshold value (the decision level).

Reliability: The method's capacity to maintain both accuracy and precision.

Sensitivity: The ability of a test to detect the presence of a particular clinical problem using a defined threshold limit (the decision value).

Specificity: The ability of a test to identify those who do not have a particular problem using a defined threshold limit (the decision value).

Standard deviation: A statistical term for describing variation in a data set (SD = square root of the variance).

Variance: A means of describing the amount of scatter in a data set.

☐ Sources of variation in the testing process

The reliability of laboratory results depends on understanding and controlling the sources of error or bias that can enter the testing process. Just as important are preanalytical factors, which can contribute as much variation to the result as analytical factors can. Many clinicians tend to think of test errors as being primarily attributable to problems with the testing process, but we have seen this isn't necessarily true. In Part I, we emphasize that proper patient preparation, collection procedures, and protection of the specimen are essential to reliable test results.

As we've said, when testing goes into the physician's office, he or she becomes responsible for the precision and accuracy of test results. The following case study of glucose testing demonstrates some potential problems the office laboratory may encounter with the new, self-contained testing systems.

CASE STUDY: GLUCOSE MONITORING WITH REAGENT-STICK TECHNOLOGY

The availability of simple methods to measure blood glucose with a visual reading or with an inexpensive meter has radically changed the management of diabetes. Experience with these methods demonstrates some of the potential problems with completely packaged reagents and what might be called black-box technology.

Evaluating the precision and accuracy of this methodology has generally been done two ways: either by repeating the test several times with the stick technology and comparing the coefficient of variation (CV) with that of standard methodology or by splitting patient specimens and comparing the results from the stick with standard methods.

The CV for blood glucose done on standard laboratory equipment is about 2%; that for a reagent stick glucose is about 18% when read visually, or 10% when read with a meter.[1] The variation of comparative results using the split sample method* was 5% to 30% when reflectance meters were used and 5% to 20% when the reagent-stick results were read visually.[1]

There was a measurable difference between the proficiency of physicians, nurses, and patients in performing these tests.[1,2] Although the reagents are completely prepackaged and the equipment is termed self-checking and self-adjusting, the technology and the person doing the test are both sources of variation. For purposes of discussion, we will divide these into variation due to instruments, methods, reagents, and the individual doing the test.

INSTRUMENT-PRODUCED VARIATION

Photometers. Many laboratory instruments are filter photometers or spectrophotometers. They measure the color produced in a chemical reaction and then compare the color with a standard; the result is expressed quantitatively. These instruments are subject to problems related to instability of the electronics. Over time, the instrument's calibration may drift, requiring recalibration. It is good laboratory practice to recalibrate the

*[Xreag − Xref / Xref x 100] where Xreag = results produced by reagent sticks and Xref = result produced by standard methods

instrument with a standard each time a group of tests is run. If many tests are done at the same time, you may need to check the calibration one or more times during the testing.

Electronic drift can be due to several factors. When the instrument is first turned on in the morning, it usually requires a warm-up period to heat the electronic components before it becomes stable. Consequently, an instrument should not be used until it is fully warmed up. Another problem is power fluctuations. Most power supplies are not entirely stable, and voltage fluctuations of several percent are common throughout the day. Inexpensive photometers are quite sensitive even to small fluctuations, but more expensive and elaborate instruments minimize their effects by internal systems that sense and compensate for them. Drift can also occur because of the light bulb's aging, the deposition of metallic material on the inside of the bulb, or dirt on the optics.

Photometers measure color reactions that take place in test tubes or cuvettes. Most cuvettes, especially those used in inexpensive systems, are somewhat variable in size and shape. This variation can cause errors in measurement. In addition, the cuvettes' optical quality may vary because of scratching or dirt on the surface. The photometer's optics may cause measurement errors.

Several factors can introduce nonlinearity to a chemical reaction's measurement. Nonlinearity is defined as the deviation from a linear quantitative relationship between the concentration of the material being measured in a chemical reaction and the instrument reading. It is common laboratory practice to calibrate an instrument with two standards (usually high and normal) and to assume that there is a linear chemical reaction over the entire concentration range being measured. If the reaction is nonlinear, this assumption is not valid.

Among the factors that influence linearity are the optical filters. Those that isolate a very narrow light wavelength produce more linear results than less expensive filters that isolate a wider wavelength. In addition, certain photodetectors produce more linear results than others. If the amount of color being measured by the instrument is too light or too dark the measurement will be nonlinear.

Because each test method has an optimal range of linearity, it is necessary to dilute the sample during the testing procedure when values exceed the range. For this reason, methods designed to measure adult bilirubin are not applicable for measuring that of neonates.

Centrifuges. Errors can also be traced to miscalibrated centrifuges. Hematocrits produced by slow microhematocrit centrifuges will be erroneously high.[3] Speed and time of centrifugation for producing plasma for coagulation tests is also of great importance. If the centrifugation is too slow or if it is not done long enough, too many platelets remain in the plasma. This erroneously shortens the apparent prothrombin or partial thromboplastin time.

Temperature errors. Enzymatic reactions and coagulation procedures are especially sensitive to temperature variation. A 7% change in activity results with each Celsius degree change. If the reaction temperature varies from that specified for the test, results will be erroneous.

METHOD-INDUCED VARIATION

Specificity. Some methods are more specific for the material being tested than others. Glucose, for example, can be measured by a variety of methods. The oldest is based on the oxidation-reduction reaction, in which glucose acts as a reducing substance. Serum contains many other reducing substances, however, and methods based on this principle overestimate the amount of glucose. More specific methods depend on enzymatic reactions. Reagent strips for glucose use the enzymatic reaction; Clinitest urine glucose test tablets measure all reducing substances.

Interfering materials cause errors in several ways. Vitamin C is found in measurable quantities in the urine of about half the population, for example.[4] It is a potent reducing substance and causes a false-positive Clinitest reaction. It also inhibits enzymatic reactions in some urine glucose dipsticks. Some urine dipstick manufacturers have recently responded to this problem by changing their formulations to minimize vitamin C inhibition.

Bilirubin also interferes with some chemistry tests, and developers of test methods usually take great pains to reduce its effects. Turbidity due to hyperlipidemia interferes with almost all photometric measurements. In severe instances, it will falsely elevate most chemical tests and hemoglobin measurement. In such cases, hematocrit is preferred over hemoglobin measurement because it is not sensitive to hyperlipidemic interference.

Technologic advances have markedly improved laboratory precision. One example of this is blood cell counts. Electronic counters, for example, measure many cells, and counting errors with these instruments are in the range of 2% to 3% for values in the normal interval. On the other hand, counting chambers can hold only a small number of cells so that variation in cell distribution can cause errors in the range of 15% or more when a normal number of cells are present. Along the same lines, mechanical pipettors are much more accurate than manual methods.

REAGENT-CAUSED ERRORS

Reagent problems are a major source of variability and error in lab testing. The purity of chemicals used is extremely important. In some cases, materials may vary from manufacturer to manufacturer; in others, there are no adequate standards for purity, as is the case with bilirubin standards. With the laboratory's increasing reliance on prepackaged reagent systems, lot-to-lot variation in manufacturing can produce erroneous results if there is no system to identify and correct such problems. In systems where reagents are prepared or reconstituted in the laboratory, the person doing this (essentially completing the manufacturing process) may need special training in order to ensure proper functioning of the machine-reagent system.

OPERATOR-INDUCED VARIATION

As we noted in Chapter 10, the quality of laboratory testing depends on the quality of the individuals involved in the process. Good laboratories and poor laboratories use the same equipment, the same reagents, and the same supplies. The major difference between a good and a poor laboratory is the personnel who take care of the machines and perform the tests.

In the case study described at the beginning of this chapter, most of the identified variation came from the person doing the test. The technology is *not* inherently less precise in one method or another; trained laboratory technologists using the same test systems can produce data with comparable or better variability than that from standard methods on standard equipment. Again, the difference lies in the people. This emphasizes the need for adequately training the staff and, when possible, using personnel with formal laboratory training (Chapter 10).

REFERENCES

1. Shapiro B, Savage PJ, Lomatch D, et al: A comparison of accuracy and estimated cost of methods for home blood glucose monitoring. *Diabetes Care* 1981;4:396.

2. Birch K, Hildebrandt P, Marshall MO, et al: Self-monitoring of blood glucose without a meter. *Diabetes Care* 1981;4:414.

3. Idaho Department of Health and Welfare: An analysis of Idaho private physician laboratory facilities and testing activities through on-site inspection, 1978.

4. Young DS: Effect of Vitamin C on laboratory tests. *Lab Med* 1983;14:278-282.

☐ Minimizing error: General considerations

We suspect that most physicians think of laboratory errors in terms of processing problems. But in actual fact, a substantial fraction of errors occur elsewhere: in patient preparation, specimen collection and handling before testing, specimen identification, and accurate result reporting (Table 17-1). And as we said in the preceding section of this chapter, the reliability of test results also depends on understanding and controlling the sources of error or bias that enter into the testing process. The office laboratorian must be aware of factors that might introduce bias or error because of methods using specimens not extensively found in other settings, such as capillary blood from a finger stick.

As we mentioned before, the physician is responsible for the appropriateness of the procedure and for test precision and accuracy in the office setting. To assume this responsibility safely, the practitioner must be sure of the following elements:

- that a quality assurance program is in place to ensure the reliability of test results
- that testing is processed in an orderly, reproducible fashion in a setting where environmental variation will not affect the result
- that all extraneous variables are excluded
- that records are available to document these facts.

TEST REQUESTS AND SPECIMEN COLLECTION

Tests should be ordered on a request form that includes the patient's name and a unique identifier, the time of collection, and the nature of the specimen. It is good practice to keep a log (not looseleaf) of all specimens collected, including the time of collection and, in the case of bacteriologic specimens, the source of the specimen. All tubes must also be marked with the patient's name and unique identifier, preferably at the time and place of collection. This is particularly important in the office setting where the tests of various family members (including some with the same first name) may be in process at the same time.

Written criteria should be established for unsatisfactory specimens, including what should be done if the name or identifier on the request slip does not match that on the specimen (it's usually best to collect a second specimen if at all possible). Protocols should be established for keeping the specimen (when appropriate) to reprocess should questions develop later. Most serum chemistries remain stable for at least seven days in the refrigerator or a month if frozen although a frost-free freezer with periodic warmups can adversely affect the stability of many analytes. Anticoagulated whole blood is stable in the refrigerator for up to 24 hours.

TEST PROCESSING

The temperature in the testing environment as well as in refrigerators, freezers, incubators, water baths, and dry baths (heating blocks) involved in testing or storing reagents or media should be monitored daily, and the results recorded. If storage conditions for reagents or media are disturbed, as in a power outage with immunohematology reagents, the reagents must be discarded as unreliable even though the expiration date has not yet been reached.

All media and reagents must be labeled with the date received and the date opened. It is obviously prudent to use the oldest dated reagents first to minimize outdating. As we noted, some materials may have to be discarded before the expiration date if the environmental storage problems develop. All working solutions should be labeled when they are prepared and the expiration date written clearly on the label if appropriate. Remember that stock solutions kept properly in storage will have a different useful life span than derivative working solutions.

For reliable results, all microscopes, centrifuges, chemistry analyzers, and other laboratory equipment must be properly maintained. The details of preventive maintenance for each piece of equipment can be found in the manufacturer's manual and is discussed in other sections of this chapter. In taking responsibility for the validity of the test information produced in the office laboratory, the physician must insist on having a log that keeps track of maintenance, problems found, and any corrective action taken. Remember that refrigerators, freezers, incubators, and heating baths or blocks are a class of equipment that can directly affect test reliability and should thus be included in the general maintenance program.

Small pieces of equipment, such as pipettes, should be stored or marked in such a way that there is little chance of inadvertently using the wrong size (for example, an RBC pipette instead of a WBC pipette), and damaged pieces should be discarded. The pipetting and diluting step is one of the most critical in many procedures and requires extreme care on the operator's part.

Among the other topics we will discuss in this section are these: 1) the necessity for written procedures for each service performed and for the operator to have a way of telling whether a procedure is working correctly, and 2) the need for explicitly written guidelines describing when a result should not be reported but analyzed a second time. Again, records must be kept of all problems and corrective actions taken. Finally, as a way of documenting test accuracy, the physician will probably want to participate in a proficiency testing program of some kind. National programs are available, but an alternative approach might be to use one in conjunction with the local hospital to ensure the comparability of test results in the two patient-care settings.

PROCEDURE MANUALS

As another way to enhance the day-to-day comparability of test results, each test procedure—patient preparation, specimen collection, and processing—must be standardized. This is usually done by having a written procedure, which the physician reviews periodically, right in the work area for each service performed.

Comparing two methods

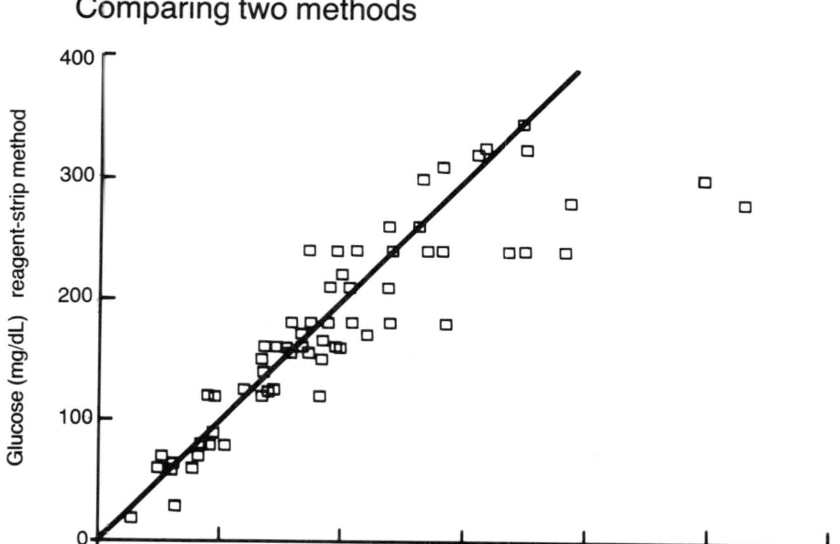

This chart compares blood glucose determinations obtained by a reagent strip method and by a conventional laboratory method and standard equipment on a split sample of the same specimen. If there were good correlation between the two, the plotted results would cluster on the diagonal line of identity.

In addition to detailing methodology, the procedure should include patient preparation information and correct specimen collection and handling, including preservatives, anticoagulant, or required special handling.

The procedure should tell how to prepare all standards, reagents, or controls (including the source of supply and the catalog number) and give step-by-step details of the method. It should describe how results are derived, any necessary calculations, the reporting units, the linearity limits, and what action should be taken when these limits are exceeded. The reference interval should be listed here as well as on the patient report (since methods and thus normal values may change from time to time). In the case of bacteriology tests, it is appropriate to detail the analytic approach to identification and to give the operator guidelines as to when assistance is required for complete identification of the organism. Finally, the procedure manual should list criteria for immediate notification of the supervisor or physician.

NEW METHOD EVALUATION

When new methods, or new lots of reagent or media are used, it is customary for the laboratory to document that the new is comparable with the old. To do this, most labs run split specimens with both old and new concurrently. Results can then be compared graphically (Figure 17-4) and statistically to assess bias between the two methods. Statistical analysis can determine the coefficient of variation (CV) of the average difference (CV) with the following formula:

$$\text{Equation 1: CV} = \frac{\text{SQRT} \left(\dfrac{\text{SUM of } (y_1 - y_2)^2}{n(n-1)} \right)}{\text{mean } y_1}$$

y_1 = results from the old reagent lot (or method)

y_2 = results from the new reagent lot (or method)

The following formula (two-sided t test) can then be used to determine whether the difference of the means is significant:[1]

$$\text{Equation 2: t} = \frac{(\text{mean } y_1 - \text{mean } y_2)}{\text{SQRT (SQRT } s^2)}$$

$t\pm$ = t value (to be used with table of t values distribution, which is available in most standard statistics texts)

s = standard deviation of the average difference

$$= \text{SQRT} \left(\frac{\text{SUM of } (y_1 - y_2)}{n\,(n-1)} \right)$$

The physician or someone designated would be responsible for reviewing these results and determining whether they are comparable without changing the reference range, whether the method requires further evaluation, or whether it can be accepted if the reference range is changed.

VALIDATING DAY-TO-DAY TEST PRECISION

Process control is also essential for precision and reliability in testing. Such a program must be built on the rock of documenta-

Quality control chart

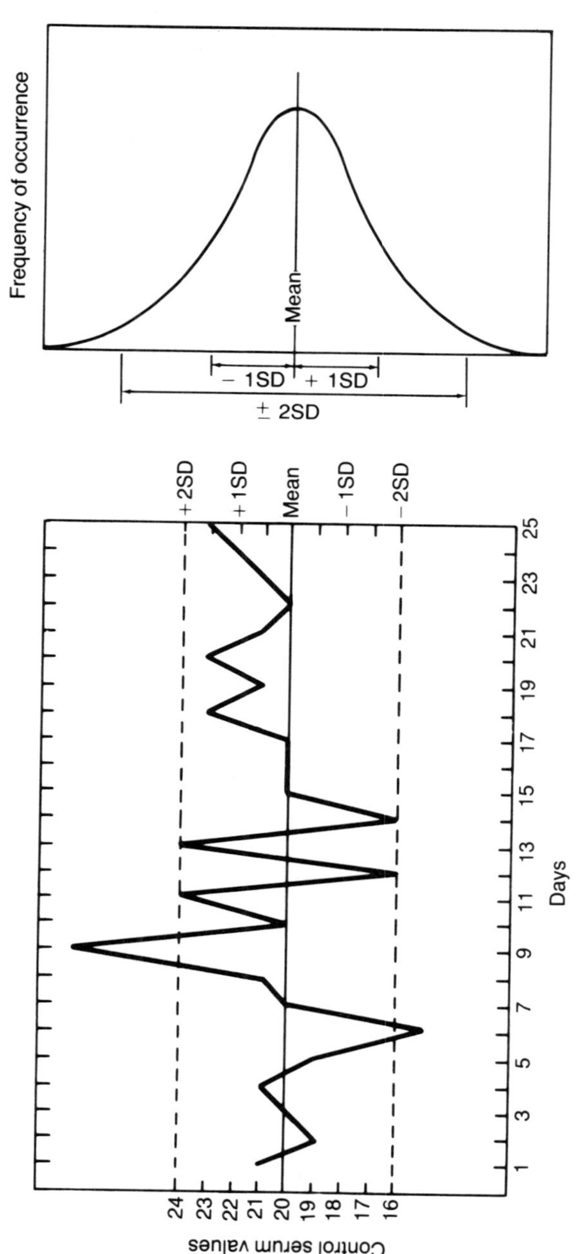

The chart at left plots individual results of a control serum's repetitive analyses; at right is a representation of the expected frequency distribution of results with this serum.

tion: detailed written procedures and a preventive maintenance program that promotes reproducible and reliable test results. But this is inadequate to ensure that the testing system, including the operator, is functioning properly on a day-to-day basis. Consequently, it is important to have a way to monitor the testing system and to provide early warning of problems that could otherwise lead to erroneous results. This important issue is discussed in detail in Chapters 12 through 16 and in a later section of this chapter.

VALIDATING TEST ACCURACY

The office laboratory should use proficiency testing programs or their local equivalent to show that its test results are comparable to those produced elsewhere in the community, region, or country. This approach does not have the timeliness of the validation methods introduced in the previous section because the results must be collated with those of other laboratories testing the same material, a process usually requiring several weeks. But this approach does document that the laboratory has been producing common coin—results comparable to other laboratories performing the same test. Although evidence of problems in processing don't come to the physician's attention until well after the fact, it is a secondary check on laboratory proficiency.

STATISTICAL METHODS AND CONTROL CHARTS

Most laboratories use both graphic and statistical methods in trying to control analytic variation of tests amenable to quantitative analysis. Potential problems often become apparent more rapidly this way. Data from sequential analysis of the same control sample may be plotted on a chart to produce a graphic display of performance. The quality-control (QC) chart (Figure 17-5) usually includes the expected mean and tolerance limits defined with horizontal lines. With this tool, it is possible to appreciate potential problems even when the control values are within tolerance limits. For example, if a series of 10 consecutive QC results fall on the same side of the mean, the operator should begin to suspect a problem (perhaps a shift in the test's operating characteristics) even though no results actually fall outside the acceptable range. Days 15 through 25 in the figure illustrate this point.

ACCEPTABLE LIMITS OF VARIATION

A variety of approaches to controlling tests amenable to quantitative analysis have been developed. The physician's office lab probably will not have the computer power necessary for some of the protocols used in today's larger labs. It will thus be important to develop easy-to-follow criteria that are clinically and economically sound and sensitive enough to give early warning of potential testing problems. Remember, too, that these criteria must then be applied to each analyte being tested.

QC IN MEDICALLY ISOLATED SETTINGS

The new self-contained testing systems that feature simple operation and stable instruments and reagents offer greater testing capability in remote areas. Many of these regions have been unable to support laboratory systems in the past.

As we stress throughout this chapter, a quality assurance program is necessary for producing reliable results, and consultation and the use of reference laboratories offer other ways to solve analytic system problems.

The clinical importance of these new testing systems is potentially greatest in just those areas where professional laboratory support is lacking. This means there is even greater pressure to keep the systems functioning reliably, and this requires still more emphasis on preventive maintenance and on day-to-day QC or results validation. Because of the isolation, the people responsible for the operation, maintenance, and repair of the systems will likely have little background in laboratory medicine. And they may have minimal training opportunities. They will, of necessity, require much more self-education of the type we discuss in the section dealing with troubleshooting. The issues are basically the same as in other settings, but like all frontiersmen, the people in more remote laboratories will have to be self-taught and, to a great extent, self-reliant.

Quality assurance programs in geographically and medically remote labs must begin with acquiring the right technology. The durability, stability, and reliability of instruments, reagents, and media for these settings must be high. An essential system component is the adequacy of written operating and troubleshooting guides and, when all else fails, the availability of dealer, manufacturer, or professional lab support for on-site troubleshooting. If a nearby practitioner is considering similar instruments or testing systems, cooperative purchasing makes good economic sense and offers operational advantages, particularly with cross-coverage in case of a system malfunction that cannot be promptly corrected.

In isolated areas, a stringent preventive maintenance program is essential for identifying potential malfunctions before breakdown or using erroneous results in patient care. Similarly, with limited access to reagents and culture media, it becomes even more important to monitor refrigerator and freezer temperatures to ensure reagent integrity and to check new shipments for maximum expiration dates.

Procedure and safety manuals are just as—or even more—important in these laboratories, providing standards and specifics for each procedure. Someone must periodically compare the way procedures are actually performed with the description in the manual. If significant changes have occurred, revalidation is necessary to make sure that comparable results are being produced. These laboratories should participate in a proficiency testing program, as a way of recognizing potential problems.

REFERENCE

1. Bermes EW, Erviti V, Forman DT: Statistics, normal values and quality control, in Tietz NW (ed), *Fundamentals of Clinical Chemistry.* Philadelphia, WB Saunders, 1976.

☐ Maintaining equipment

Testing accuracy and precision depend on having equipment that works right when you need it. Two important considerations in selecting instruments, then, are these: reliability and the availability of technical support in case of machine malfunction or breakdown. Most laboratorians also subscribe to the idea that the risk of malfunction or breakdown is minimized by a periodic preventive maintenance program.

Such a program begins, of necessity, when the new instrument or system arrives in the laboratory. Even before it is unpacked, the people responsible for its installation and operation are duty bound to become familiar with the instruction and operator's manuals. Each piece of equipment should have a file that includes manuals, the names and phone numbers of local sales and service people, warranty information, and an equipment information log to record routine maintenance, problems, corrective actions, and the dates involved. Using the manufacturer's manuals as a guide, you should also develop a schedule of suggested preventive maintenance for each instrument. Here are some pointers for equipment found in most laboratories.

Refrigerator. Used to store reagents and media plates, the laboratory refrigerator should have a freezer unit, and the temperature should be checked and recorded daily. This is done with a thermometer sitting in a pint-sized bottle of water on the top shelf of the refrigerator. An acceptable temperature range is between 4° and 8° C. This necessary procedure provides validation that reagents and media have been maintained at an appropriate temperature before use (exposure to elevated or freezing temperatures can prematurely degrade many such preparations). A refrigerator requires little maintenance except for cleaning the motor's filter and periodic defrosting if it is not a frost-free model. Food and drink should never be kept in the lab refrigerator, both for employee safety and for the purity of the chemicals.

Incubator. This relatively simple device is a box with a heating element and a thermostatic control. It is designed to keep its interior at a constant temperature, usually 37° C for most microbiology work. Many incubators have a hole in the top where a thermometer can be inserted to monitor the internal temperature without opening the door. If this is not possible, the incubator thermometer should be placed in a rubber-stoppered, pint-sized bottle filled with water, and the temperature should be checked at least daily, recorded, and the thermostat adjusted, if necessary. The incubator temperature should be maintained within 1 C of the desired value since even small changes can dramatically affect the isolation of some pathogens.

Centrifuge. These instruments are used to spin down microhematocrits, prepare urine sediments for microscopic examination, and separate serum and plasma from blood. It is self-apparent that running them faster or slower than designated for preparing the microhematocrit or urine sediment will produce an inaccurate result. Similarly, inadequate centrifugation of clot for serum preparation may produce anomalous results, particularly if a serum separator tube is used and the serum is held for later processing. The manufacturer's instructions must be followed carefully, particularly with reference to centrifuging with a balanced load. The instrument should be set on a stable counter top and operated only with the lid closed until the centrifugation is complete. Never use pencils, fingers, hands, or anything else to slow the centrifuge; this can hurt the equipment or the operator. Clean the inside of the bowl daily with a bactericidal solution and after any sample spills.

Check the centrifuge speed periodically, record the results, and correct any variance from the specified speed range. Commercial laboratory repair services or consultants from a local reference laboratory will perform this service for a fee. The check should be done at least semiannually, more frequently in high-volume laboratories.

Microscope. This precision instrument requires a certain amount of care to function properly. Dust and dirt are everywhere and can cause trouble in both the mechanical and optical components. Although surfaces exposed to dust are also accessible to cleaning, such "cleaning" doesn't help the glass surface, so it's best to cover the microscope with a hood or keep it in a cabinet. In most cases, you can use a grease-free brush or a frequently washed, absolutely dust-free linen rag and distilled water (easily produced by breathing on the surface) to clean the outer lenses. If an organic solvent is absolutely necessary for cleaning the outer surface of the ocular or objective lenses, use a very small amount of alcohol. Only the manufacturer or a qualified service representative should clean the mechanical parts or re-grease and clean the optical system, preferably once a year.

Refractometer. The specific gravity (relative density) of a fluid may be determined with a refractometer (an instrument determining the refractive index of a substance). These instruments must be periodically checked with distilled water and with solutions of known dissolved solid concentration (usually a saline solution). The refractometer can be adjusted accordingly.

Coagulation analyzer. Coagulation tests done in the office lab will probably be analyzed with a fibrometer. Check the manufacturer's manual for a maintenance schedule. The mechanical or electrical timing devices should be checked periodically, and the optical or electrical sensing elements must be kept clean.

Blood chemistry analyzer. Most of these instruments have a built-in colorimeter or reflectometer and use premeasured reagents in kit form. The colorimeter operates by passing a beam of light through a tube or cuvette containing the specimen and reagents and measuring the absorption of specific parts of the light spectrum. A reflectometer operates by analyzing the reflectance of specific parts of the light spectrum from a reagent-impregnated pad or film to which the patient specimen has been applied.

The degree of absorbance or reflectance, as measured at a specific wavelength, is a function of the concentration of the analyte being tested. Daily, weekly, and monthly preventive maintenance, as recommended by the manufacturer, is essential to the instrument's working properly. Daily maintenance, after an adequate warm-up, may include cleaning and a calibration check. Periodically, the cuvette should be inspected and the instrument checked for linearity and stray light. Keep the manufacturer's customer service phone number or that of a local service representative for ready reference.

Because of the complexity and cost of these instruments, it might be worthwhile to have a service contract for regular maintenance and repair. But be sure to ask about the availability and accessibility of service personnel before entering into such an agreement. Such contracts can be cost-effective, however, by precluding unexpected expenditures for parts and service calls (usually $50 an hour or more, door-to-door from the service center) and minimizing downtime and lost revenue.

Other instruments. Timers and stopwatches should be checked periodically, and it's easy to do against a standard time source like the telephone time message. Urinometers are notorious for being miscalibrated; and for this reason, we do not recommend using them.

☐ Validating day-to-day precision and accuracy

Different types of testing systems require different approaches to validation. The reliability of hematology and chemistry test results, for example, is most often checked with control materials that allow statistical analysis of result validity. This doesn't work in microbiology, however, where individual components and materials are regularly checked to make sure they give appropriate answers. Specific details of quality assurance for each discipline can be found in Chapters 12 through 16. We discuss more general aspects of day-to-day result validation in this chapter.

A written quality-control (QC) program should include defined limits of acceptable performance, a written record that the program is operating, evidence of corrective action when results exceed tolerance limits, and a daily review by the supervisor and monthly one by the physician.

Written evidence of the program's operation, corrective actions, and periodic review are extremely important because of the physician's responsibility for result validity (Chapter 7). This in no way diminishes the importance of other aspects of the overall quality assurance program including the need for rigorous patient identification routines and other issues we've discussed elsewhere in this chapter.

Another aspect of process control requires a senior staff member or the physician to review all test results. The physician, of course, is in an ideal position to identify results that don't seem to fit with the patient's condition. If the specimen has been preserved, the test can be reprocessed or sent to a reference lab for confirmation. In many hospital laboratories, this may be the most timely way to identify potential problems.

HEMATOLOGY

As we said, we check the validity of these procedures with control materials that simulate the specimen being tested. Such a program can be built on commercially prepared controls with known values or on retesting patient specimens (useful only for some quantitative hematologic procedures). Commercial programs add to the cost of the test, but the comparisons they offer are valuable: You can compare your results with those of other lab-

TABLE 17-2

Is the test system functioning properly?

Determine the coefficient of variation of the average differences used to find out

	y_1	y_2	$y_1 - y_2$	$(y_1 - y_2)^2$
1.				
2.				
3.				
:				
:				
:				
n.				
Sum				

y_1 = the value from day 1

y_2 = the value from day 2

SQ RT = Square Root

n = the number of paired sera or bloods

$$\text{Mean} = \text{the average value of the total data set} = \frac{\text{Sum } y_1 + \text{Sum } y_2}{2n}$$

$$\text{Coefficient of variation (average difference)} = \frac{\text{Sq Rt [Sum } (y_1 - y_2)/n]}{\text{Mean}}$$

oratories using the same method-machine combination and also, to a lesser extent, get some idea of the bias of these methods compared with the same material processed on standard laboratory analyzers.

You can validate all hematology parameters except platelets and peripheral smear results by retesting patient specimens. Specimen deterioration causes but negligible changes in these values,[1] so any difference exceeding the interassay variability is probably due to problems with the machine or method. The results of tests performed one day can be reprocessed at the beginning of the next day, after the instrument is warmed up and calibrated. Then determine the coefficient of variation (CV) and whether the means are significantly different using the statistical methods described by equations 1 and 2 in the third section of this chapter. Table 17-2 shows an easy way to determine the CV of the average difference. Any variance exceeding the preset limits should suggest potential problems with the methods. This approach has two major defects: You cannot become aware of problems with the methods or equipment until the following day (when significant differences of individual patient results should be reported to the physician and a new report issued), and it lacks the feature of comparing results produced by other laboratories.

COAGULATION

This testing poses somewhat different problems. Lack of standardization of some reagents makes it difficult, at times, to produce universally constant coagulation results. In the situation we're discussing, it is particularly important to have such constancy between the physician's office and the hospitals where the patients may be hospitalized. Thus splitting patient specimens and comparing the two sets of results may be the most practical quality assurance program.

Commercial controls are also available for coagulation testing, but they have a couple of serious problems. First, they may introduce a factitious bias because of their formulation; and second, they come in lyophilized form and require the laboratory to reconstitute them by adding a critical amount of reagent grade water. For these reasons we do not recommend this approach for most physicians' office labs.

CHEMISTRY

Several approaches can be used to document result validity. Each offers advantages and disadvantages as to cost and operational considerations.

The first approach involves using the patient's specimen within the office laboratory. In fact, most laboratorians would recommend that any abnormal result or any result greater than a predetermined difference (delta check) be reprocessed in the lab before reporting the result. This adds some expense and requires that the laboratory have access to earlier results either from their own records or from the patient's medical record.

Another approach is to reprocess the specimen in a local reference lab. The drawbacks here are a loss of timeliness and a serious erosion of the referring laboratory's professional and financial position. In addition, by referring only presumably abnormal specimens, the physician may not recognize anomalous normal results that are, in fact, abnormal.

Rather, it is preferable to develop programs that will better ensure the quality of the office laboratory test result. We described one good way in the discussion of QC for hematology tests; it is based on the fact that the concentration of most analytes in serum will be stable if the specimen is stored in a refrigerator at 4 C. The results of tests performed at various times during one day can be used to detect variation that exceeds preset limits, prompting the operator to evaluate potential problems. As we said, however, the operator may not become aware of problems until the following day when significant differences in one patient's results should be reported to the physician and a new report issued.

Patient specimens can also be used as the basis of a quality assurance program in which excess serum—either from one patient or pooled from many patients—can be sent to a reference laboratory to assess all analytes the lab processes. Aliquots of this control serum can then be run daily for each analyte (more frequently if the volume justifies it) and the control results compared to the assayed value. If results exceed predetermined values, they should be questioned and the machine and methods checked to identify the problem or provide a basis for confidently issuing the results. Two major advantages of this QC method are that office lab results would be correlated with those of the reference lab and that actual levels tested would depend on the sera and would vary from week to week. This approach provides analyte levels that are close to critical clinical decisions—and that's where process control is most important.

Excessive handling of patient specimens has some inherent problems, too—specifically an increased risk of hepatitis for the lab employees. The reference laboratory could provide their own QC sera with analyte values close to the medically important levels. This is a more costly approach, but the information it provides seems worth the expense. In addition, it is an opportunity for the office laboratorian to develop consultation resources to help deal with troublesome methodology or machine problems, an essential service for someone who has no specific training or experience in laboratory medicine.

Since not all office chemistry methods have appropriate commercial controls, this may be the only QC method available for some labs. An important part of using controls of this kind is to cross-validate the control material by running the old and the new control concurrently for a few days. And again, it is important to have predetermined limits of acceptable performance with guidelines on what to do when the controls are out of limit. This approach also helps employees gain a sense of the variance in the office laboratory over time, as we've mentioned.

Over the last few decades, QC programs have developed that are based on commercially available stabilized control sera with analyte concentrations at or near critical decision levels. This has played an important role in improving the quality of clinical chemistry results in big, automated laboratories. These materials (with human or animal serum as a base matrix) are supplied in liquid or lyophilized form and have analyte concentrations adjusted to bring them to critical decision levels. Because many chemistry methods use enzymes from nonhuman species, there is an expected difference among results produced by different methods and machines that does not necessarily translate directly into differences in using the methods on human serum specimens. Although this material lets laboratories control a wide range of analytes and evaluate method precision, the bias can pose a problem in evaluating accuracy.

To improve the usefulness of these commercial controls, broad programs have been developed with many participating laboratories and with computers comparing results by machine-method combination. This lets the laboratorian document that the exhibited bias is a result of the material and not the method being used in the particular laboratory. It also allows estimation of the test result variance over time and some comparison of one lab's variance with comparable facilities. Unfortunately, such programs are applicable to only a small fraction of physicians' office testing, but we hope manufacturers will soon develop appropriate materials and programs for that setting.

MICROBIOLOGY

Unlike chemistry and hematology, this discipline does not lend itself to the mathematical QC approach—repeat analyses of control specimens. But quality assurance is no less necessary in dealing with microorganisms' many forms and metabolisms. Consequently, QC in microbiology focuses on validating the reagents and media used to identify microorganisms and evaluating their antibiotic susceptibility. A most important aspect of a quality assurance here is a careful definition of how much evaluation the laboratory can do and the development of consultative resources for help with problems beyond its ability. Details of quality assurance for specific microbiology tests are discussed in Chapter 14.

Media. Since microorganisms are generally identified by their growth and biochemical reactions on various types of media, it is of utmost importance that the media perform properly. Inoculating plates from the current lot with known stock organisms is one way to check on the medium's ability to support growth of potential pathogens and to validate that biochemical reactions are working right. Culture media should also be checked for sterility to make sure that contaminants are not confused for pathogens. Before using media in patient testing, the laboratorian should check to be sure that plates are smooth, adequately hydrated and the media is not dried or loosened from the sides of the container or tube.

Stock organisms. Reference cultures can be maintained in the office laboratory or in a reference laboratory and used to check media, reagents, stains, and susceptibility disks. The number and nature of the organisms required will depend on the extent of the services offered and the specific media and materials used in the evaluation of microorganisms in the office lab.

Other procedures. Serologic procedures, such as coagulase, catalase, and oxidase determinations that are used to identify pathogens, should be processed with appropriate positive and negative controls. Stains should also be checked weekly and whenever a new batch is started with known gram-positive and gram-negative organisms to make sure they will identify these organisms. If such special stains as Ziehl-Nielson are used, check to make sure they will stain the organisms appropriately. Because stained slides produce qualitative and not quantitative results, they should be stored for easy retrieval and review should questions develop in the future.

Susceptibility testing. An important aspect of modern microbiology is evaluating the susceptibility of potential pathogens to antibiotics. In large laboratories this is most often done by using paper disks impregnated with varying drug concentrations. Since clinicians frequently use this information in selecting antibiotic therapy, it must obviously be reliable. The disks, first, should be used only with single isolates or pure cultures (this is true for the A disk to give presumptive identification of a group A beta-hemolytic streptococcus). The disks should be stored according to the manufacturer's recommendation and checked periodically for their activity with stock cultures with known susceptibility patterns. In the office laboratory, where a single cartridge may be used over a number of days, the potency of the disks should be checked at least weekly.

SEROLOGIC AND PREGNANCY TESTING

Control of serologic and pregnancy testing is somewhat analogous to that required in microbiology because many control materials are not standardized. But it is nonetheless important to include daily process controls to validate that these complex procedures are operating appropriately. Manufacturers often provide positive and negative controls, but the titer of the positive control is frequently so high that it is insensitive to even large changes in the test's operating characteristics. Consequently, it is incumbent on the office laboratorian to validate the titer of the positive control and, if necessary, dilute it with an appropriate diluent to make it more sensitive to methodologic problems. For example, if the antibody in a pregnancy test has deteriorated but the control had remained positive through a 32-fold dilution when tested with the intact antibody, it's obvious that the test's diagnostic capability could be severely compromised while the control still gave the expected positive result.

IMMUNOHEMATOLOGY (BLOOD BANK) PROCEDURES

These should not be attempted in the office laboratory unless done by a qualified laboratory technologist and unless appropriate licenses have been secured.

REFERENCE
1. Brittin GM, Brecher G, Johnson CA, et al: Stability of blood in commonly used anticoagulants. *Am J Clin Pathol* 1969;52:690-694.

☐ Troubleshooting out-of-control results

So far, our emphasis in reducing laboratory error has been on primary prevention—a quality-control (QC) program to minimize the risk of erroneous results and a preventive maintenance program to minimize the potential for system malfunction or breakdown. But we cannot entirely avoid equipment malfunction, and the QC program can raise questions. If a QC result is outside preset limits (or "out of control"), for example, we may have a problem of system integrity that requires immediate investigation. Out-of-control values can result from malfunction or misuse (human error) of one of the following components:

- instruments,
- standards,
- controls,
- reagents.

A MILLIGRAM OF PREVENTION IS WORTH A KILOGRAM OF CURE

Many out-of-control results can be avoided, and as we said, prevention is probably the best way of doing it. But if you don't have a good preventive maintenance program, the way to investigate a problem must include a check of all the preventive steps that should have been taken.

To be effective in identifying and correcting problems flagged by out-of-control QC values, personnel must become thoroughly acquainted with what happens at each step of a normal run. By being observant and noticing color and volume changes, the speed of mechanical steps, and instrument sounds, the operator may catch abnormal conditions when they occur. This perception is often all that's necessary, and it is by far the easiest way to find the cause of out-of-control results. Once the problem is identified, correcting it is usually straightforward.

To learn what happens at each step, the operator should be taught by an experienced technologist. Otherwise, it's the more difficult matter of self-education—being observant, studying instruction manuals, and using other materials such as this book. It is important for the operator to understand the nature and characteristics of the methodology being used. If someone knows only that the specimen and reagent are put in a tube, there's a color change, and it's read in an instrument, troubleshooting an out-of-control result will be impossible. The ability to diagnose test problems quickly is the difference between a well-educated, experienced technologist and someone with less training and insight.

PREVENTIVE MAINTENANCE

Because effective preventive maintenance precludes many out-of-control situations and because the first step in troubleshooting is to review it, we will start by briefly reviewing its various aspects.

Instruments. Before running a test, you should make sure that the instrument is in top operating condition. Preventive maintenance must be done on a regular schedule, with some checks made yearly and others made biannually, quarterly, monthly, weekly, or daily. Make a list of functions to be checked and parts to be cleaned for each instrument after studying the instruction manual that comes with it. If less-than-daily maintenance has been performed on schedule and if the daily maintenance is performed before running the test, the chances of malfunction during the run are minimal. Conversely, if preventive maintenance is not routinely practiced, the possible causes of an out-of-control result are mountainous rather than molehillish.

Every instrument consists of one or more systems, each of which has its own checkpoints. Let the instruction manual and your experience be your guides in setting up a preventive maintenance schedule. Some suggestions that are impractical for maintenance may be quite useful in troubleshooting certain malfunctions. Many of the newer instruments' instruction manuals have very thorough preventive maintenance and troubleshooting sections. The suggested schedules should obviously be followed as closely as possible.

Optical systems. Checking the cleanliness of lamps, filters, and lenses is important. Many optical instruments such as filter photometers provide kits for periodic checks on sensitivity and linearity, wavelength calibration, and stray light. These kits suggest when to change or clean lamps, clean filters and lenses, or check other parts of the optical system.

Cuvettes, which are usually packaged as a component of the reagent kit, are a most important part of the optical system. In order to read the test reaction accurately, cuvettes must be clean, dry, free of scratches, and properly aligned in the cuvette well. Some systems have reusable or flow-through cuvettes. They must be clean and without scratches, and you should keep a supply of new ones to replace the old. It is also important to maintain a supply of spare lamps for quick replacement.

Electronic and electrical systems. There is little to do in the way of preventive maintenance of electronic systems. Electronic components do not deteriorate gradually, and there is no way to check or replace them before deterioration causes a problem. They are either functioning or not, and it's obvious when they aren't. On some instruments, the zero point should be checked periodically and reset if necessary. At least three spare fuses should be kept in stock for each fuse in your instrument. If one blows, it can be replaced immediately. If it blows again, however, find out why before replacing it. Most instruments require a period of electronic and thermal warmup before stable, reliable readings can be made.

Temperature control systems. Any temperature-controlled instrument must have its temperature checked before each run. It should be recorded at least once daily.

Fluid measurement systems. Measuring systems range from small disposable, plunger-type pipettors to pumps and sophisticated devices in some of the electronic blood cell counters. As we've said before, mouth pipetting is hazardous and must be prohibited. If a glass pipette is used, a hand-controlled vacuum bulb should be used with it. Visually check the pipetting devices you use each day for creeping, setting, or leaks. Changes in calibration and reading of standards and controls may also indicate miscalibration of the pipettor.

Standards are to be treated with the greatest respect. This includes keeping them tightly capped; storing them at the proper temperature; examining them for discoloration, precipitates, debris, and growth of organisms each time they are used; being careful to avoid contamination; and discarding them on or before the expiration date. Before starting to use any new standard, compare it in a run with the old standard to be sure it gives equivalent values. The run must include controls to assure that the system was in control when the standard was checked. Make a notation in the QC records that the standard was put into use, the check was made, and the standard was satisfactory. Whoever makes the check should date and initial the notation.

Controls must be reproducible. Thus when reconstituting lyophilized material, be sure that pipettes are the right size, in good condition, clean, and properly used and that the distilled water is chemically pure and uncontaminated. The control must also be properly mixed and usually left to stand for a time before use. It should be kept capped and refrigerated, and some must be used shortly after reconstitution. The reproducibility of alkaline phosphatase, for example, may be acceptable only if the control is run between two and four hours after reconstitution. At least two controls, a normal and an abnormal, should be used in each run. Before using a new lot, check it in a run with the old one. This way, an in-control value on the old lot assures that the system was working properly when the new lot was started. Make a note to this effect in the QC records, with the date when you started the new lot.

Reagents. A new reagent must be checked in the system just as controls and standards are. It should be run with standards and controls that were used with the old reagent system. QC records should indicate the date that new reagents were checked and found acceptable. Treating reagents as respectfully as standards and controls can help prevent out-of-control results.

Human preventive maintenance. Don't do tests that are beyond the competence and education of your employees. Before they do a new one, they must receive adequate training in the method. This includes reading manuals and methods and, if possible, performing the test under the supervision of someone who is experienced with it.

Although clerical errors are difficult to avoid, a carefully planned system can make people aware of where to look for them. Label and check are key words in the laboratory:

- Every reagent should be clearly labeled and the label checked whenever it's used.
- Every specimen container should be labeled with the patient's name or other identification. When transferring part of a specimen from one container to another, check the names or numbers against each other to make sure there's no mix-up.
- When recording results, check the name or number on the container with the name or number on the worksheet. Never assume that the name on the next container is the same as the next name on the worksheet.

Out-of-control analysis form

Test _______________ Instrument _______________ Date _______ By _______________

I. Clerical check

	Reading	Conversion (including calculations)
Initial		
Check		

DRY RUN

II. Instrument settings

	Abs/Conc	Rate/Term	%T/OD	Other	Factor	Filter/Wavelength
Your procedure						
SOP						

III. Cuvettes

	Condition - All cuvettes			Individual			Flow-through	
				Brand	Size	Matched	Leaks	Plugs
Your procedure						1 read 2 read		
SOP	Clean	Free from scratches	Aligned properly			Within 1%T	None	None

IV. Procedure (reverse side)

WET RUN

V. Standards/Controls/Reagents

	Accepted value	Out-of-control value	Repeat cont/std	New cont/std	New reagent	New reagent	New reagent	In-control value
Standard								
Control								
Low point								
Midpoint								
High point								

Cause of out-of-control value: _______________________________

____

Date _________ Reviewed by _________ Position _________ Comments

Section head

QC coordinator

Pathologist

(Back)

IV. Procedure

Constituent in order added	Constituent 1	Constituent 2	Constituent 3	Constituent 4	Constituent 5	Constituent 6
Your procedure						
SOP						
Appearance of constituent						
Your procedure						
SOP						
Expiration date of constituent						
Your procedure						
SOP						
Volume added						
Your procedure						
SOP						
Measuring device used						
Your procedure						
SOP						
How was it used*						
Your procedure						
SOP						
Mixing operation used/adequate?						
Your procedure						
SOP						
Reaction time						
Your procedure						
SOP						
Reaction temperature						
Your procedure						
SOP						
Time lapse before reading						
Your procedure						
SOP						

*If pipette, rinse out, blow out, drain, point-to-point; if automatic, was it functioning well, poorly, any leaks or plugs?

BRINGING OUT-OF-CONTROL RESULTS INTO CONTROL

We estimate that adhering to the preventive maintenance measures we've described will avoid at least 75% of out-of-control results. The remainder can usually be identified by following a systematic approach. The worksheet (Figure 17-6) is a guide to such an approach. This systematic troubleshooting has several major steps: 1) a dry run to detect deviations from standard procedure; 2) an equipment examination to detect malfunction; 3) if these don't reveal the error, repeat the test to check standards, controls, and reagents.

First of all, it is important to recognize the out-of-control situation. This is usually through the use of control samples that give a result outside acceptable limits. Other indications are standards or patient values outside the expected range.

Once it has been determined that the test is out of control, the first step should be to review clerical procedures, including specimen identification, and to recalculate results.

Next, do a dry run of the test, comparing each step with the written procedure. Pay special attention to using the right reagents, volumes, incubation times, intervals between readings, wavelength settings, other instrument settings, and the order of adding reagents. Examine the bottles of reagents, standards, and controls and the tubes used in reading the test results. Are they the right color? Is there any turbidity or precipitation? Are test-tube volumes right? Is the color of the liquid in the tube the shade and intensity that you expect? Are the reagents, standards, and controls within the expiration date or past it?

Check the equipment. Are all pipettors and other measuring devices working properly and giving correct volumes? Are the temperatures correct? Does the photometer perform correctly with the calibration kit? Have you checked the cell counter aperture for partial obstruction? Has there been any problem in the last several days?

If you still haven't found the cause of the problem, check the test data. Are controls, standards, and patient values all giving unexpected results? Are both controls giving unexpected results or only one? Is the control too high or too low? Is it giving a value that is exactly half or double the accepted value?

If it is necessary to repeat the test, run an old and a new

standard and an old and a new control along with your patient. If one of these is giving false values it will be quite apparent.

Problems with one or more of the controls is likely if the standards give expected readings and if the patient values are in their usual ranges. The standards may be at fault if controls and patient values are proportionally altered. If you can't get valid readings for standards, controls, and patients and the instrument appears to be functioning properly with the calibration kit, this suggests a faulty reagent system. To check reagents, it is best to start with a new, unopened kit. Do the test again, with all new reagents, controls, and standards.

Reviewing QC records can sometimes give a clue to the deterioration of a component in a test system. Look for gradual loss of control with both the normal and abnormal control samples. This is a clue to reagent or instrument deterioration. If, on the other hand, a trend is seen with one control but not the other, the fault may lie with the control materials. An abrupt change that coincides with a change in reagent, control, standard, or instrument quickly suggests the source of the problem.

Some out-of-control situations appear to be refractory to troubleshooting. It may help to bring in an outside consultant, such as an experienced medical technologist, who can provide the dispassionate observation needed to solve the problem. Once the solution is found, write a complete report to be kept on file in the laboratory. Such records can be helpful for future troubleshooting and can provide ideas for additional preventive measures and in-service education.

☐ Record keeping

In most aspects of medical practice, the physician can evaluate the quality of work the ancillary staff does by observing it directly. This is not true of laboratory testing. Although the physician makes important medical decisions based upon his assumption that lab work is accurate and precise, he has no direct way of judging its quality. It is therefore very important to have good records of the laboratory's work and procedures. They can help the physician determine how much he or she can trust the work being done.

Record-keeping requirements are very strict for hospital and independent laboratories. They should be no less so for the physician's office lab. The malpractice and liability implications of complete records are discussed in Chapter 7.

DEFINING THE NEED FOR RECORDS

There are a number of reasons why the office lab should keep good records. First is that physicians should be able to demonstrate that their laboratories do work of comparable quality to larger facilities. Quality-control (QC) records can offer this assurance by demonstrating excellence of work.

Second, if the physician were involved in a malpractice suit that questions the quality of lab work done in his or her office, it will be very important to be able to produce records demonstrating acceptable QC, proficiency survey performance, and staff competence.

Third, there appears to be a trend toward licensing regulations for physicians' office labs. Several states already require them to be licensed, and more are probably considering it. The kind of records we will discuss in this chapter are usually a requirement for laboratory licensure.

PERSONNEL RECORDS

Personnel with varying levels of training, experience, and competency do tests in doctors' offices, and it is important to document certain information carefully. Employment records should detail the person's training and level of certification—the length of training in laboratory procedures, whether the program was accredited, whether the individual has been certified by a national certifying agency, and if so, which agency. A copy of the certificate and registration number would be helpful should verification be necessary. This becomes especially important if accuracy is questioned after the person who did the test has left the doctor's employment.

For people who are trained on the job, it's wise to document the training, including a demonstration of skills that require patient manipulation, such as venipuncture. Continuing education activities for the office staff should also be recorded.

QUALITY CONTROL

One of the basic QC tenets is this: "If it isn't written down, you can assume it wasn't done." No matter how carefully work is performed and how well QC procedures are adhered to, no one can judge the quality of the work if records are inadequate. QC documentation has several components: First are daily logs that record standardization and control values run each time a test is performed. These are best kept as a worksheet along with the results of patient tests. These sheets should be signed and dated by the person doing the tests. It's also important to calculate variance of daily QC testing. The limits for acceptable performance should be determined periodically, and the daily control specimen results should be judged against these standards.

In most states where doctors' office laboratories are licensed, laboratory personnel must run periodic proficiency test samples and report results to the accrediting agency. Many laboratories also subscribe to proficiency test programs from a professional organization. The physician should review these proficiency test results and daily QC records—and document that he or she does so. If results are outside acceptable limits, there should be evidence of corrective action.

Other quality-control records include evidence of periodic temperature checks, such performance checks as centrifuge calibration, and equipment maintenance and repair records.

RETAINING RECORDS

Federal regulations and rules of the College of American Pathologists and Joint Commission on Accreditation of Hospitals indicate that laboratory records, including QC records, daily logs, and records of standardization and equipment surveillance should be kept for at least two years. It would be a good idea for physicians' office laboratories to observe similar retention times (Table 17-3).

PROCEDURE MANUALS

As we discussed in the third section of this chapter, this manual should have detailed instructions for each procedure the laboratory uses. In the case of such common procedures as blood

Suggested guidelines for keeping laboratory records and materials*

Reports	3 years
Quality-control records	3 years
Log books	1 year
Maintenance records	As long as the instrument is in use
Bone marrow reports and slides	25 years
Special blood study reports and slides	25 years
Routine blood smears	10 days
Routine plasma and serum	7 days

*Adapted from: *Guidelines for Professional Practices in Pathology.* Skokie, Ill., College of American Pathologists, 1983.

counts, the manual can merely refer to a standard textbook and page where it can be found. For tests that use kits or packaged reagents such as dipsticks, the package insert is considered adequate. Again this word of caution: Manufacturers occasionally change package insert instructions. It's important to have the most up-to-date in the notebook.

It is good practice for the physician to review this manual annually and to document that it was done. Directors of hospital and independent laboratories have to follow a similar procedure, and it is evidence that the person responsible is aware of the laboratory's procedures and has approved them. It also helps ensure that no unauthorized changes or shortcuts have been taken.

Many of these record-keeping chores may look like overkill, but each has been found to be important. There is every reason for doctors with office laboratories to insist on the same level of performance validation and documentation found in licensed and accredited laboratories. QC documentation is invaluable when test results are called into question.

REFERENCES

1. *Standards for Laboratory Accreditation.* Skokie, Ill., College of American Pathologists, 1982.

2. Carlson DJ: Some proposed accreditation standards for small medical laboratories. *Lab Med* 1982;13:661-665.

Choosing tests for in-office analysis

The decision to run a particular laboratory test in your office should be made like any other patient management or business decision: in an informed, thought-out, organized way. Among the factors to be considered are medical needs, technical ability to do the test, the adequacy of personnel, legal restrictions, financial considerations, managerial considerations, and physician and patient convenience. We'll consider them in turn.

Medical needs. Certain test results may be particularly helpful during the patient's visit in order to diagnose a problem quickly or initiate or revise therapy. Tests for proteinuria are an accepted essential part of a prenatal visit, for example. Tests for bacteriuria will allow early therapy in a patient who may have cystitis. Theophylline concentration is helpful in adjusting dosage in patients who are getting an inadequate therapeutic effect from the drug. In other instances, epidemiologic considerations may suggest doing a test in the physician's office. Examining urethral discharge for gonococcus, for example, may permit early therapy and reduced exposure of uninfected individuals.

Technical factors. This may be the major consideration in your decision-making process. First and foremost: Can the test be done accurately in the office laboratory? Do you already have competent personnel who can do the test, or must you train or recruit someone with the necessary skills? Will the office staff require professional supervision to perform the test, and will that supervision be available whenever the testing is needed? How easy is it to perform the test? If the test requires the technician's full attention, will this interfere with office routine? Does the test make the technician unavailable to assist you for too long? Is the test easy enough to be run by another staff member if the technician is out?

Another consideration is whether the specimen can be transported to another laboratory without deteriorating in transit. Specimens for sedimentation rate and prothrombin time must be tested within 16 to 24 hours after being drawn, and the specimen must be refrigerated. If there is no other laboratory facility in town and if the patient cannot travel to another laboratory, you may have no choice about performing these tests in your office.

Before deciding on one test, you should consider whether another test might give the same information. Is it necessary, for instance, to do a red cell count if hemoglobin or hematocrit are already available? What is the preferable method for measuring urine specific gravity? Do you want to use a urinometer, a refractometer, or a reagent stick?

Equipment availability is also a consideration. If you are going to measure serum enzymes, you should have a spectrophotometer that can make measurements in the ultraviolet range and record and calculate rate reactions. If you have a simple colorimeter for glucose measurements, for example, you may have to buy additional equipment to perform enzyme measurements but not urea tests.

Another technical consideration is the workload you anticipate. This can affect your decision in a number of ways. For example, a technician must perform any test fairly often in order to remain proficient. Another reason for considering workload is that all reagents have a finite life expectancy. Your workload should be great enough to use almost all of the kit's reagents before they expire. It is not economically or technically desirable to do tests with too low a workload.

Finally, you must consider certain safety factors. Special safety hoods are necessary when performing tests that involve noxious solvents. And it requires special precautions to handle virulent, highly infectious organisms. Some tests, such as the benzidine method for occult blood, use carcinogenic reagents, and these methods should not be used in an office laboratory.

Legal considerations. A number of states require licensing doctor's office laboratories, but they usually exempt those that have fewer than a certain number of practitioners. In a few states, however, any office laboratory doing even the simplest test, such as dipstick urinalysis, must be registered and fulfill certain requirements such as participating in an approved proficiency program. California recently enacted legislation requiring all doctor's offices receiving reimbursement under the MediCal (that state's Medicaid) program to be staffed with licensed medical technologists who are graduates of a four-year medical technology program and have passed a state licensing examination.

The other legal consideration is malpractice exposure, which we discussed at length in Chapter 7. As with all medical procedures, there is a malpractice risk in performing and reporting laboratory tests for which the office staff is untrained, inexperienced, or unqualified. Physicians have been held responsible for properly interpreting and using test results from a reference laboratory. But when the analysis is done in the office laboratory, the physician is responsible for the technical accuracy of the tests as well. Evaluating a professional negligence problem involving the office laboratory would probably involve the same state-of-the-art standards that apply to a pathologist-laboratorian in the same situation.

Financial considerations. Although income production may not be the primary motivating factor in this decision, it is certainly a consideration. With all kinds of tests, the daily volume has a direct influence on the cost. Cost per test must include the costs of reagents for standardization and quality control, out-dating wastage, proficiency testing, equipment amortization, salaries, and space. Because many of these are fixed costs that are unrelated to test volume, they can be a significant factor when volume is low. Front-end questions to consider include whether you'll need additional equipment or space. If you are setting up a new test, will the technician need to be trained? Will there be a charge for it, and will a replacement be necessary during the training? An introduction to laboratory cost accounting is discussed in Chapter 8.

Other financial considerations are the cost of the test if an independent lab does it, the price you can charge for it, and third-party reimbursement policies and fee schedules. In some states, for instance, third-party payers will pay according to the

Should you do the test or send it out?
Some issues to consider

Medical
 Immediate diagnosis or therapy
 Epidemiologic needs

Technical
 Ability to perform the test accurately
 Availability of an alternate test
 Need for new equipment
 Patient transportation
 Specimen transportation
 Staff competency
 Supervision
 Workload for proficiency
 Workload for economy

Legal
 Licensing
 Malpractice hazard
 Personnel certification

Financial
 Cost to patient
 Independent laboratory charges
 Need for patient return visit or phone call
 Needed space
 Needed equipment
 Third-party reimbursement policy and fees
 Your per-test charge

Managerial
 Availability of consultation, staff training, supervision, trouble-shooting

lowest charge for the test from an independent laboratory (Chapter 6).

Managerial considerations. With simple tests, the technician can frequently follow the instructions in the kit and get a high level of proficiency, accuracy, and precision. With more complex tests, your technician may need supervision or consultation. You should also consider the likelihood of needing help in troubleshooting problems with the test.

Physician and patient convenience. There is no question that it is convenient to have laboratory results during the patient's visit. Immediate results allay anxiety in both physician and patient. And with certain patient populations, there are even more significant benefits in having the results available quickly. Some patients are elderly or infirm, or live at such a distance that a return visit or a special trip to the pharmacy is inconvenient and impractical. For the physician, another visit or calling the patient or the pharmacy can be a poor use of the clinician's time, which may require an additional expense to the patient.

How to judge laboratory tests. For each test you are considering, it may be useful to prepare a checklist that rates each factor we have discussed. Table 18-1 shows a sample worksheet.

19

Using reference laboratories and consultation

In parallel with deciding whether or not to perform a test in your office, you may decide to send certain tests to another laboratory. This chapter discusses how to select that facility. There are two basic steps in the process. First, you must define your requirements for a reference lab. Then you must evaluate each lab's ability to meet your needs.

DEFINING REQUIREMENTS

Make a list of the tests you are likely to refer to an outside laboratory. Your choice may vary according to whether the list consists mostly of high volume, routinely performed tests or such specialized tests as endocrine or immunologic procedures.

Service considerations may be important. Turnaround time, starting with when you obtain the specimen and ending with when you get the report in your office, may vary markedly from one lab to another. This depends on when and how often specimens are picked up, when tests are done, and how and when you get the reports. Some labs provide daily or more frequent pickup service. Others require you to mail specimens in containers they supply. Some will accept an unprocessed whole blood specimen, while others require you to centrifuge and separate the plasma before submitting it for testing. You should decide which method best suits your practice. Is it necessary for the referral laboratory to supply containers, or are you willing to provide them? Will you need stat testing? If so, can you deliver the specimen to the laboratory, or will it have to be picked up?

Consultation and interpretation needs must be defined. Will a laboratory that provides accurate and timely test results be enough, or do you want to be able to consult a laboratory professional about choosing appropriate tests and interpreting results? Do you want to work with a laboratory that gives you advice and assistance, helping you choose tests and test methods and assisting with trouble-shooting and quality control?

Reporting method and format may also be important. Some laboratory reports are more readable and informative than others. You may have a format preference. Reports can be returned to your office several ways: messenger, mail, printing terminal, or telephone for urgent reports. These are factors to consider in your choice.

EVALUATING THE LABORATORIES

Table 19-1 shows a checklist for evaluating reference laboratories. This section will elaborate on some of its points.

Scope of tests. Does the laboratory offer the tests you need? It is conceivable that you may occasionally ask for tests the laboratory does not provide. In such cases, will it send the specimen to another laboratory that can do the test? It is inconvenient to have to deal with several laboratories.

Specimen handling. Does the laboratory provide a manual on how to submit specimens? It should include clear instructions for specimen collection including patient preparation, type of tube or anticoagulant, special rules for preserving and shipping specimens, lists of interfering drugs or foods, quantity of sample required, special handling, such as centrifugation before shipping, reference ranges, and if possible some interpretive comments. Does the laboratory provide specimen containers, mailers, and request forms? Does it pick specimens up from your office? Is its schedule convenient? Is there a delay of more than two hours between pickup and delivery to the lab? If so, are specimens refrigerated in transit? Must blood samples be centrifuged to provide serum or plasma, or does the laboratory accept whole-blood specimens? Does the laboratory provide containers with special preservative for tests where sample deterioration may occur, such as glucose, acid phosphatase, or urine for microscopic examination?

Turnaround time and frequency of testing. How long does it usually take to get the report you need? Is this adequate for your clinical needs? Can stat requests be accommodated? What is expected turnaround time for unusual tests? You may want to ask about such tests as CEA, parathyroid hormone, and tricyclic antidepressant drug concentrations.

Reports. Do you like the report format? Look at several examples including chemistry, hematology, coagulation, and microbiology. Is it hard to find the result, the reference range, the time and date the sample was obtained? Do results of such tests as protein electrophoresis include interpretations? Does the laboratory's manual contain reference ranges, test methods, and interpretive information? How are test results returned—by messenger, printer, mail? Are significantly abnormal results reported to you by telephone? Will the laboratory give you a list of test values that would prompt a telephone report? Does the report highlight test values outside the reference range?

Consultation. Can you easily get advice from a laboratory professional concerning appropriate tests for a patient, a test result that is inconsistent with the patient's condition, or result interpretation? If you tell the laboratory a result is inconsistent with the patient's condition, do personnel get defensive? Do they offer to retest the submitted specimen or ask for a new sample for testing? Do they say it will be done without charge to the patient? Do they question you about interfering drugs or foods that may have caused the inconsistency? Will the laboratory give your personnel assistance? Can you establish a relationship with one specific laboratory professional, or do you talk to an anonymous voice at the other end of the phone when you call for advice?

Licensing and accreditation. Ask the laboratory representative if your state requires licensing. Is the laboratory licensed? If the laboratory receives specimens from outside the state, is it subject to federal inspection and licensing? Is it licensed for interstate testing under the Clinical Laboratory Improvement Act (CLIA) of 1974? Is it accredited by the College of American Pathologists (CAP) or Joint Commission on Accreditation of Hospi-

Text continues on page 297

A checklist for evaluating a reference laboratory.

	Good	Adequate	Inadequate
Scope of tests			
Appropriate range	____	____	____
Unusual tests referred to another lab	____	____	____
Specimen handling			
Adequate instruction manual	____	____	____
Specimen containers provided	____	____	____
Mailers	____	____	____
Request forms	____	____	____
Specimen pickup			
Convenient schedule	____	____	____
If two-hour delay in delivery			
Samples refrigerated	____	____	____
Whole blood acceptable	____	____	____
Special preservatives provided	____	____	____
Glucose	____	____	____
Acid phosphatase	____	____	____
Urine for microscopic	____	____	____
Turnaround time			
Adequate for routine tests	____	____	____
Adequate for unusual tests	____	____	____
Stat tests accommodated	____	____	____
Reports			
Flagging of abnormal results	____	____	____
Interpretative reports?	____	____	____
List of abnormalities prompting a phoned report	____	____	____
Method for returning reports	____	____	____
Readable format	____	____	____
Significantly abnormal results reported by phone?	____	____	____

	Good	Adequate	Inadequate
Consultation			
Advice about:			
Selecting appropriate tests	______	______	______
Interpreting results	______	______	______
Resolving inconsistent results	______	______	______
Help with your office laboratory	______	______	______
Can you establish a relationship with one person?	______	______	______
Licensing and accreditation			
Accreditation	______	______	______
CAP	______	______	______
JCAH	______	______	______
Licensed by federal agency	______	______	______
Medicare	______	______	______
CLIA	______	______	______
Licensed by state	______	______	______
Cost			
Test fees	______	______	______
Charges to your laboratory:			
Consultation services	______	______	______
Printing terminal	______	______	______
Shipping charges	______	______	______
Specimen collection supplies	______	______	______
Extra services			
Customer service representative	______	______	______
Educational materials	______	______	______
Training for your staff	______	______	______
Professional and business reputation			
Length of time in the area	______	______	______
Reputation for quality and integrity	______	______	______

Services that a laboratorian consultant might provide the physician's office laboratory.

Quality assurance
Analyze results
Design program:
   Documentation
   Parallel testing of specimens
   Proficiency testing services
Provide control materials
   Assayed values from your lab
   Economic packaging
   Precision data for your lab
   Reconstituted
Provide statistical services

Regulation and reimbursement
Advise about regulations
Alert physician to changes in rules
Assist with licensing
Inspect lab for compliance with
   regulations

Instruments and kits
Advise about:
   Equipment maintenance and
      documentation
   Equipment repair
   Group purchasing
   Leasing of equipment to lab
   New products
   Troubleshooting
   Validation of system
Evaluate product in relation to:
   Accuracy and precision of system
   Costs
   Level of personnel
   Needs

Education
Develop support group for personnel
   Formal educational programs
   Information tutorials
Provide check sample programs
Recommend newsletters for physicians
   and office staff
Train technologists to provide
   consultative services

Consultation
Advise about choice of tests
Advise about interpretation of results

Troubleshooting
Advise about procedure or system
   change
Follow-up education
Prompted by QC data
Prompted by request from office lab
Problem solving

Business consultation
Advise about fees
Advise about computer services
Analyze costs (send-out versus
   in-office testing)
Help with form design
Help with record keeping

tals? Is it inspected and accredited for Medicare reimbursement? Each of these agencies has similar requirements regarding training and experience of technical personnel, equipment maintenance, quality-control programs, proficiency testing, and safety procedures that help assure quality work.

Cost. Although independent and hospital laboratories bill patients directly in most cases, there may be differences in costs to the patient and to your office. Ask for a fee schedule, and compare prices for specific tests. Are there overhead costs to your office, such as postage or shipping costs, provision of sample containers, and such supplies as collection tubes or needles? Are there differences in how long it takes to prepare test request forms? Do they charge you for the cost of a terminal for receiving printed reports? Do they charge for consultation?

Extra services. Some laboratories provide excellent educational services such as frequently revised manuals and newsletters or training in specimen collection and handling. Will they give your staff advice? Is there a customer service representative who deals with your staff and handles service problems?

Professional and business reputation. Does the lab have a reputation for quality and integrity? How long has it operated under its present leadership in your area? How many of your professional colleagues use this laboratory?

By considering these questions for several laboratories, you will probably find significant differences between them. Some factors will be of lesser importance. Quality issues as judged by licensing or accreditation will weigh heavily in the decision.

PROFESSIONAL CONSULTATION

In addition to performing and reporting tests on your patients, the reference lab may offer other valuable services (Table 19-2). It can assist you with the cost-effective operation and quality assurance of your office laboratory, for example.

The systems currently being sold or in development give physicians' office labs the ability to do hematology, coagulation, microbiology, pregnancy, allergy, and clinical chemistry tests. The procedures are in all likelihood run by an office staff member, but the physician is ultimately responsible and liable for the quality of the test result and for correctly interpreting it and applying it to patient management decisions. The physician with little or no background in laboratory medicine should make a point of using local consultative services to evaluate the available systems, develop procedures that will provide information comparable to the high quality produced in other laboratories, and develop quality assurance protocols to ensure the accuracy and precision of the reported results.

A pathologist or laboratorian might provide help and consultative services in such areas as these:

- Evaluating the tests appropriate for the physician's office laboratory, appropriate methods, recommended equipment, laws and regulations covering operation and reimbursement for office-based laboratories, and cost analysis of in-house processing compared with sending the tests out.
- Selecting and training office staff involved in the testing process, and advice about any restrictions on using some personnel in test processing.
- Developing appropriate forms and record-keeping.
- Evaluating the equipment and testing kits being marketed for the office laboratory, including potential problems that may be encountered during evaluation.
- Developing appropriate quality assurance protocols.
- Establishing proficiency testing and specimen-based, self-testing, self-instructional programs.
- Developing a daily quality-control program—materials, statistical analysis, and appropriate records.
- Documenting maintenance and repair services and supplementary help with troubleshooting machine and method problems.
- Shared purchasing, accreditation, and other programs.
- Laboratory computer services.

There is not now a completely satisfactory system of controls for the office laboratory setting. Establishing a quality assurance program to ensure result validity is terribly expensive either in dollars or technician time, which amounts to the same thing. Ideally, the diagnostics industry will develop an inexpensive control that has no interfering substances and does not require reconstitution in the office laboratory. This could provide a material that would specifically validate the testing process at or close to critical decision levels. A joint quality assurance program run in conjunction with a local laboratory could also solve some of these problems. In fact, a good consultative relationship with a reference laboratory can serve the interests of your office, the reference lab itself, and your patients.

GENERAL REFERENCES

1. Nicholls AL: How to use the reference laboratory, American Society of Clinical Pathologists Technical Improvement Service 13:59-63; 14:66-71; 15:50-61, 1973.

2. Shaw ST: Selection of reference laboratory services. *Clin Lab Med* 1983;3:509-523.

Chemistry analyzers and supplies for physician's office laboratories

A. Capillary blood glucose systems

COMPANY	PRODUCT	NOTES
Ames Division, Miles Laboratories	Glucometer and Dextrostix	Dry-chemistry whole-blood analyzer uses Dextrostix test strips and a reflectance photometer
Ames Division, Miles Laboratories	Visidex	A test strip for glucose monitoring in whole blood
Boehringer Mannheim Diagnostics	Chemstrip bG	Dry-chemistry whole-blood test for glucose determination
Lifescan	Glucoscan Plus	A blood glucose monitoring system with dual-beam optics; it includes test strips, control, and meter

The authors have tried to make these listings as complete as possible. Because of the number of products available and being developed daily, however, they realize that it's impossible to be comprehensive. Readers should therefore understand that an omission implies nothing about a product nor does inclusion mean an endorsement.

B. Dry-chemistry systems

COMPANY	PRODUCT	NOTES
Ames Division, Miles Laboratories	Seralyzer	Dry-chemistry system based on cellulose strip
Boehringer Mannheim Diagnostics	Reflotron	Whole-blood dry-chemistry system that uses a reflectance photometer
Eastman Kodak	Ektachem DT60	Analyzer that uses dry-film technology
Syntex Medical Diagnostics	AccuLevel TDM	Noninstrument-based enzyme immunoassay

C. Electrolyte test systems

COMPANY	PRODUCT	NOTES
AVL Scientific	Electrolyte analyzer	Uses whole blood to determine sodium and potassium by an ion-selective electrode (ISE)
AVL Scientific	Blood gas analyzer	Whole-blood analyzer
Boehringer Mannheim Diagnostics	LyteTek 1000	Measures potassium from whole blood by ISE; includes all reagents
Corning Medical	Electrolyte analyzers	Several fully automated small analyzers for sodium, potassium, chloride, calcium, pH, and carbon dioxide
Electro-Nucleonics, Inc.	Starlyte	Whole-blood analyzer; uses ISE for sodium and potassium
Mallinckrodt	Na/K analyzer	Flame photometer for sodium and potassium
Nova Biomedical	Nova electrolyte analyzers	Several whole-blood analyzers for calcium, potassium, calcium, carbon dioxide, chloride, and pH

| Orion Research | Electrolyte analyzers | Several whole-blood analyzers for sodium, potassium, calcium, chloride, and pH |
| Phytec | Versalyte II | Whole-blood ISE analyzer for sodium and potassium |

D. Fecal occult blood detection systems

COMPANY	PRODUCT	NOTES
Ames Division, Miles Laboratories	Hema-Chek	A rapid slide test
Helena Laboratories	ColoScreen	Slide test
SmithKline Diagnostics	Hemoccult	Slide test

E. Pregnancy test systems

COMPANY	PRODUCT	NOTES
Baker Instruments	Pregnancy test	A rapid slide test for quick determination
Diagnostic Technology Hybritech	b-HCG Check Tandem-Visual HCG	A urine hCG test Measures hCG in urine and serum by a tube method of enzyme immunoassay
ICL Scientific Monoclonal Antibodies	Slide pregnancy test Pregnastick	Measures serum or urine Measures hCG in serum and urine by enzyme immunoassay
NMS Pharmaceuticals	Nimbus	Rapid sensitive test using serum or urine in a colorimetric assay
Organon Teknika	Duoclon slide test, Pregnolisa, Pregnospia, Pregnosticon Dri-Dot	A variety of tube and slide tests to detect hCG in urine and serum
Quidel	Quest	Measures hCG in serum or urine by enzyme immunoassay with a monoclonal antibody

Roche Diagnostic Systems	Pregnosis, Sensi-Slide, Sensi-Chrome, Sensi-Tex Placentex	A variety of slide and tube tests
Ventrex Laboratories	Ventrescreen HCG	Enzyme immunoassay for qualitative determination of hCG in serum and urine; includes controls
Wampole Laboratories	UCG-Beta Slide Monoclonal, u-hCG Lyphotest, u-hCG Beta Stat	Slide and tube tests to detect hCG

F. Urinalysis test systems and supplies

COMPANY	PRODUCT	NOTES
Ames Division, Miles Laboratories	Multistix	Multiparameter test strips
Ames Division, Miles Laboratories	Tek-Check	Strips for preparing urinalysis QC material
Boehringer Mannheim Diagnostics	Chemstrip 9, Chemstrip 7, others	Multiparameter test strips
Clay Adams	Sedi-Stain	Premixed stains for urinary sediment
EM Diagnostic Systems	Urintrol	Urinalysis QC materials
ICL Scientific	Kova	System has slides, pipettes, controls, tubes to standardize concentration, and stain for microscopic exam
V-Tech, Inc.	Count-10	System includes slides, tubes for standardizing concentration, and stain for microscopic exam

G. Wet chemistry systems

COMPANY	PRODUCT	NOTES
Abbott Laboratories	Vision	Novel, highly automated whole-blood analyzer
Bio-Analytics	Smart Alex II	Semiautomated instrument for a wide range of chemistry tests and immunoassays
Bio-Analytics	Uno 1 test kits	Reagents for the Smart Alex II
Boehringer Mannheim Diagnostics	Chem System 400	Test tube system that includes instruments, reagent, standards, and controls
Boehringer Mannheim Diagnostics	Unilab	Test tube system that includes rack and pipettes
Boehringer Mannheim Diagnostics	Unimeter 330K	Test tube and dry-chemistry system that includes instruments, reagents, standards, and controls
Boehringer Mannheim Diagnostics	Unitest	Test tube and dry-chemistry system that includes an instrument, reagents, standards, and controls
CooperBiomedical	Request	An automated, random-access analyzer with a small computer. Reagent kits, standards, and controls are also available
CooperBiomedical	Assist	A fully automated system programmed for 40 tests; it includes reagents and controls
CooperBiomedical	Demand	A fully automated, high-speed, random-access system for larger group practices

CooperBiomedical	Analyzer II Plus	A semiautomated system programmed for 40 tests; it includes reagents and controls
Corning Medical	Magic	Immunoassay system for hormones
Electro-Nucleonics, Inc.	Gemstar	Automated system with reagent kits
Electro-Nucleonics, Inc.	Gemeni	A centrifugal fast automated analyzer with reagent kits
EM Diagnostic Systems	UniPak 500	Wet-chemistry system
EM Diagnostic Systems	UniPak 100	A single-beam mini-analyer
General Diagnostics	Test kits	Reagent systems for a range of chemistry tests
Gilford Instrument Laboratories	Stasar	Semiautomated spectrophotometer
Gilford Instrument Laboratories	Supplies	Reagents and controls for common chemistry tests
Ilex	Prompt	Automated whole-blood system
Mallinckrodt	Serometer 370	A test tube system with kits
Mallinckrodt	Serometer 375	Same as the 370 with five more measurements by UV spectrophotometer
Mallinckrodt	Serometer 380	Same as the 375 with a small computer for faster output
Mallinckrodt	Gran-U-Chem	Prepackaged reagents in granular form
Phytec	Versamate I Versamate A	A simple, manual system A semiautomated system
Sclavo	Uni-Fast	A semiautomated analyzer and reagent system

SenTech	ChemPro 1000	Novel fully automated system; uses a disposable cartridge
Sequoia-Turner	Analyte 350	A general-purpose spectrophotometer-fluorometer with calculation for all areas of the lab
Seragen Diagnostics	Quick-Chem	A test tube system that includes reagent kits, standards, controls, incubator, and calculating colorimeter
Turpen Laboratory Systems	ATAC 2000	Semiautomated system for a variety of chemistry tests and immunoassays

GENERAL EQUIPMENT AND SUPPLIES FOR PHYSICIANS' OFFICE LABORATORIES

COMPANY	PRODUCT	NOTES
American Scientific Products	Medifuge	Table-top centrifuge
American Scientific Products	Touch mixers	For mixing samples in test tubes
American Scientific Products	Tube rocker	Mixer for blood and urine samples
Ames Division, Miles Laboratories	Aliquot mixer rotator	A mixer for hematology, chemistry, and serology applications
Boehringer Mannheim Diagnostics	Centrifuges	Table-top models
Clay Adams	Dynac II	Table-top centrifuge
Damon, International	Spinette	Table-top centrifuge
Equipment Company Drucker	Centrifuges	Table-top models

HEMATOLOGY ANALYZERS AND SUPPLIES FOR PHYSICIANS' OFFICE LABORATORIES

A. Blood cell counters and supplies

COMPANY	PRODUCT	NOTES
American Scientific Products	Sysmex analyzers	Blood cell counters that range from three- to eight-parameters
Baker Instruments	Series 130	A three-parameter cell counter (RBC, WBC, and hemoglobin) that uses 40 μL of blood
Baker Instruments	Series 150	A five-parameter cell counter (RBC, WBC, MCV, hemoglobin, and hematocrit) that uses 40 μL of blood
Boehringer Mannheim Diagnostics	Hemo-W	A small system for WBC and hematocrit
Boehringer Mannheim Diagnostics	M430	A system for WBC, RBC, hemoglobin, and hematocrit
Clay Adams	QBC	Novel blood cell instrument that uses hematocrit and fluorescent-stained buffy coat to measure RBCs, WBCs, and platelets
Clay Adams	QBC Plus	An updated QBC that includes seven chemistry tests
Coulter Electronics	Model S-Plus, $S^5 50$, $S^7 70$, others	Systems range from red and white cell counters to many parameters
Diagnostic Technology	Picoscale	A four-parameter system (WBC, RBC, hemoglobin, and platelets)

General Diagnostics	Sicklequik	A rapid qualitative test to detect the presence of and distinguish between heterozygous and homozygous sickle cell hemoglobin
Mallinckrodt	Profile 700, Model 390, others	A range of cell counters
Phytec	Versacount	Three-parameter analyzer (RBC, WBC, hematocrit)
Sequoia-Turner	Cell-Dyn systems	A range from simple to complex cell counters
Seragen Diagnostics	Quick Count, Quick Count/Plus 2	Two- and four-parameter counters (WBC and hemoglobin plus RBC and hematocrit)

B. Coagulation test systems and supplies

COMPANY	PRODUCT	NOTES
American Scientific Products	Supplies	Cups and pipette tips to use with the Fibrometer
BBL Microbiology Systems	Fibrometer	Coagulation timer that measures PT, APTT, and thrombin time with a moving electrode that detects a clot in the plasma mixture
Boehringer Mannheim Diagnostics	Du 500	A compact coagulation system that measures PT and APTT
CooperBiomedical	Coagulation products	Kits for APTT, PT, and fibrinogen; controls are also available
Diagnostic Technology	Supplies	Hematology standards, controls, and a QC program

Company	Product	Notes
General Diagnostics	Coag-a-mate 150	A single-channel, semiautomated instrument with reagents for PT, APTT, and fibrinogen
General Diagnostics	Coag-a-mate 2001	A semiautomated system for PT and APTT
General Diagnostics	Reagents	For the Coag-a-mate systems
Helena Laboratories	Dataclot	A timer for PT and APTT
Logos Scientific	Elvi 818 Digiclot	A timer for PT, APTT, and thrombin time
Medical Laboratory Automation	Electra 750	A timer for PT, PTT, and thrombin time
Ortho Diagnostic Systems	Coagulation products	Included are reagents for PT, APTT, thrombin time, and fibrinogen

---

C. Sedimentation rate systems and supplies

COMPANY	PRODUCT	NOTES
Acculab	Sediplast	An erythrocyte sedimentation rate (ESR) system including a rack and disposable tubes that use 0.8 mL of blood
American Scientific	ESR system	A Westergren system including rack and tubes
Becton Dickinson Vacutainer Systems	Sedirak	Wintrobe tube rack
Chase Instruments	Sed rate system	Rack and tubes included
Coulter Electronics	Zeta sedimentation rate system	Rapid capillary tube system based on zeta potential; it includes an instrument, tubes, and interpretation charts
Ulster Scientific	Dispette	A disposable, self-filling Westergren sed rate system

IMMUNOLOGY ANALYZERS AND SUPPLIES FOR PHYSICIANS' OFFICE LABORATORIES

A. Immunology test systems

COMPANY	PRODUCT	NOTES
American Dade	Rheumatoid Factor Test	Latex agglutination slide test to identify rheumatoid factor (RF) in serum
CooperBiomedical	Immunology kits	Kits for immunoglobulins, RF
Diagnostic Technology	Latex slide tests	Tests for antinuclear antibodies, RF
ICL Scientific	Rheuma-Fac	Latex agglutination slide test for RF
ICL Scientific	RID assays	To determine immunoglobulins and serum proteins
Organon Teknika	Rheumanosticon Dri-Dot	A rapid test for qualitative and quantitative determination of RF in serum
Seragen Diagnostics	Seratest RF	A latex slide test for RF
Wampole Laboratories	Rheumaton	A two-minute latex test to detect RF
Wellcome Diagnostics	Rheuma-Wellcotest	A rapid latex test to detect RF in serum
Wellcome Diagnostics	Thyro-Wellcotest	A two-minute latex slide test to detect thyroglobulin antibodies
Wellcome Diagnostics	CRP-Wellcotest	A two-minute latex slide test to detect and semiquantitate CRP in serum

B. Allergy test systems

COMPANY	PRODUCT	NOTES
MAST Immunosystems	Allergy testing system	Tests allergen-specific Ig-E
NMS Pharmaceuticals	IgE ELISA kit	A test system specific for allergy IgE

MICROBIOLOGY ANALYZERS AND SUPPLIES FOR PHYSICIANS' OFFICE LABORATORIES

A. Culture systems and supplies

COMPANY	PRODUCT	NOTES
American Scientific Products	Gonodecten	A presumptive test for gonococcus; it uses a color reagent to detect oxidase-positive bacteria in urethral discharge
American Scientific Products	Gram stain control slides	Prepared slides for Gram stain QC
American Scientific Products	Culturette swabs	Throat culture swabs
Ames Division, Miles Laboratories	Microstix Candida	Reagent strips with selective media for *Candida*
Ames Division, Miles Laboratories	Microstix-3	Three-way reagent strips to detect bacteriuria
Bacti-Lab	Streplate	Media for throat cultures
Boehringer Mannheim Diagnostics	Unibac media system	System uses divided plates with selective media and diagnostic guides
Difco Laboratories	SpotTest reagents	Ready-to-use stains, biochemicals, and other reagents
General Diagnostics	Autobac	A growth-detecting instrument

General Diagnostics	Microbiology test kits	Biochemical and antibiotic testing reagent systems
Gilford Instrument Laboratories	Gilmed	System to detect urinary tract infection
Logos Scientific	Bacteriology stains	Premixed stains
Mallinckrodt	Gonoscreen	30-minute limulus amebocyte lysate test for presumptive diagnosis of gonococcus from urethral discharge
Marion Scientific	Culturette	Throat culture swabs and holding media
Medical Technology	Uricult, Respiracult, Biocult	Dip-slide media for urine, throat, and GC media
Seragen Diagnostics	MicroChek	Dip-slide system for urine cultures
SmithKline Diagnostics	Isocult	Prepared culture media for rapid determination of organisms
Wampole Laboratories	Bacturcult	Urine collection and culture media in the same tube

B. Immunologic test systems and supplies

COMPANY	PRODUCT	NOTES
American Dade	RPR card test	Syphilis serology tests
Antibodies Incorporated	Detect-A-Strep	Seven-minute direct agglutination test for group A beta-hemolytic streptococcus (GABHS)
CooperBiomedical	LEAP (Liposome Enhanced Agglutination Procedure) tests	Kits for strep, infectious mononucleosis (IM), others

Diagnostic Technology	Latex slide tests	For antistreptolysin-O (ASO), c-reactive protein (CRP), IM
Difco Laboratories	D.A.I. Strep A Test	A latex agglutination test for qualitative detection of GABHS from throat swabs
Hynson, Westcott & Dunning	Directigen	Seven-minute direct agglutination test for detecting GABHS from throat swabs
ICL Scientific	Latex slide tests	Agglutination tests for ASO, CRP, and IM
Marion Scientific	10-Minute Group A Strep ID	Direct latex agglutination test for GABHS
Medical Technology	Respiralex	A rapid direct agglutination test for GABHS
Organon Teknika	Monosticon Dri-Dot	A slide test to detect IM antibodies
Ortho Diagnostics	Monospot	A slide test for IM
Ventrex Laboratories	Ventrescreen Strep A	Rapid direct agglutination test to detect GABHS
Wampole Laboratories	Streptozyme	A rapid slide test to detect streptococcal antibodies
Wampole Laboratories	Mono-Test	A test for IM antibodies in serum
Wellcome Diagnostics	Streptex	A rapid latex system for qualitative detection and identification of the Lancefield group of streptococci
Wellcome Diagnostics	Wellcogen	Rapid latex tests to detect antigens to group B streptococci, *Hemophilus influenzae* b, and *Neisseria meningitides* A, C, Y, and W135

QUALITY-CONTROL PRODUCTS FOR PHYSICIANS' OFFICE LABORATORIES

COMPANY	PRODUCT	NOTES
American Association of Bioanalysts	Proficiency testing service	Proficiency testing program for small labs covers most testing areas
College of American Pathologists	Excel	Proficiency testing program for small labs covers most testing areas
Streck Laboratories	Blood cell controls	Blood cell and capillary blood glucose materials for quality control

2

Manufacturers and suppliers of office lab equipment and supplies

AVL Scientific
PO Box 337,
Roswell, Ga. 30077
(800)421-4646

Abbott Laboratories, Diagnostics Division
Abbott Park, Ill. 60064
(800)323-9100
In Illinois (312)937-2688

Acculab
50 Maple St.,
Norwood, N.J. 07648
(201)767-1600

American Association of Bioanalysts
205 West Levee,
Brownsville, Tex.
(512)546-5315

American Scientific Products
1430 Waukegan Rd.,
McGaw Park, Ill. 60085
(312)689-8410

Ames Division, Miles Laboratories
PO Box 70,
Elkhart, Ind. 46515
(800)344-9100
In Indiana (219)264-8901

Antibodies Incorporated
PO Box 1560,
Davis, Calif. 95617
(800)824-8540
In California (916)758-4400

Bacti-Lab, Inc.
PO Box 1179,
Mountain View, Calif. 94042
(800)227-7300
(800)446-8600
In California (415)968-3815

Baker Instruments Corp.
PO Box 2168,
Allentown, Pa. 18001
(800)345-3127
In Pennsylvania (215)264-2800

BBL Microbiology Systems, Becton Dickinson and Co.
PO Box 243,
Cockeysville, Md. 21030
(800)638-8663

Becton Dickinson Vacutainer Systems
P.O. Box 818,
Rutherford, N.J. 07070
(201)460-4900

Bio-Analytics
PO Box 333,
Palm City, Fla. 33490
(800)327-8282
In Florida (800)432-9608

Boehringer Mannheim Diagnostics
9115 Hague Rd.,
Indianapolis, Ind. 46250
(800)845-2000
(800)428-5074
In Indiana (800)382-5200

Chase Instruments
288 Glen St.,
Glens Falls, N.Y. 12801
(800)451-4351

Clay Adams
299 Webro Rd.,
Parsippany, N.J. 07054
(800)638-1532
In New Jersey (201)887-4800

College of American Pathologists
5202 Old Orchard Rd.,
Skokie, Ill. 60077-1034
(312)966-5700

CooperBiomedical
One Technology Ct.,
Malvern, Pa. 19355
(800)233-5505
In Pennsylvania (215)251-2000

Corning Medical
63 North St.,
Medfield, Mass. 02052
(800)255-3232

Coulter Electronics
PO Box 2145,
Hialeah, Fla. 33012-0145
(800)526-6932
In Florida (305)885-0131

Damon, International Equipment Co. (IEC Division)
300 Second Ave.,
Needham Heights, Mass. 02194
(800)225-7786
In Massashusetts (617)449-0800

Diagnostic Technology
240 Motor Parkway,
Hauppauge, N.Y. 11788
(800)645-6288
In New York (516)582-4949

Difco Laboratories
PO Box 1058,
Detroit, Mich. 48232
(800)521-0851
In Michigan (800)344-8526

Drucker Co.
3240 W. 16th Ave.,
Hialeah, Fla. 33012
(305)557-4480

EM Diagnostic Systems, Inc.
480 Democrat Rd.,
Gibbstown, N.J. 08027
(800)527-5541
In New Jersey (609)423-6300

Eastman Kodak Co.
P.O. Box 92894,
Rochester, N.Y. 14692
(800)445-6325

Electro-Nucleonics, Inc.
368 Passaic Ave.,
Fairfield, N.J. 07006
(800)631-1067
In New Jersey (201)227-6700

Fisher Scientific
711 Forbes Ave.,
Pittsburgh, Pa. 15219
(412)562-8300

General Diagnostics
201 Tabor Rd.,
Morris Plains, N.J. 07950
(800)631-8060
In New Jersey (201)540-2837

Gilford Instrument Laboratories
132 Artino St.,
Oberlin, Ohio 44074
(800)221-7527

Helena Laboratories
PO Box 752,
Beaumont, Tex. 77704
(800)231-5663
In Texas (409)842-3714

Hybritech, Inc.
11095 Torreyana Rd.,
San Diego, Calif. 92121
(800)854-1957
In California (619)455-6700

Hynson, Westcott & Dunning
Charles and Chase Streets,
Baltimore, Md. 21201
(800)638-1532
In Maryland (301)837-0890

ICL Scientific
11040 Condor St.,
Fountain Valley, Calif. 92708
(800)382-2527
In California (714)546-9581

Ilex
400 W. Cummings Park,
Woburn, Mass. 01801
(800)874-4539
In Massachusetts (617)938-3744

Lifescan Inc.
1025 Terra Bella Ave.,
Mountain View, Calif. 94032
(800)227-8862
In California (800)982-6132

Logos Scientific, Inc.
700 Sunset Rd.,
Henderson, Nev. 89015
(800)821-2495
In Nevada (702)565-1383

MAST Immunosystems
630 Clyde Ct.,
Mountain View, Calif. 94043
(415)961-5501

Mallinckrodt
P.O. Box 5840,
St. Louis, Mo. 64114
(800)645-5467
In Missouri (314)895-2271
In New York (516)567-2300

Marion Scientific Corp.
9233 Ward Parkway,
Kansas City, Mo. 64114
(800)821-7772
In Missouri (816)966-5000

Medical Laboratory Automation
500 Nuber Ave.,
Mount Vernon, N.Y. 10550
(914)664-0366

Medical Technology Corp.
PO Box 218,
71 Veronica Ave.,
Somerset, N.J. 08873
(800)526-2125
In New Jersey (201)246-3366

Monoclonal Antibodies
2319 Charleston Rd.,
Mountain View, Calif. 94043
(800)227-8855
In California (415)960-1320

NMS Pharmaceuticals
1533 Monrovia Ave.,
Newport Beach, Calif. 92663
(800)854-3002
In California (800)367-4200
(714)645-2111

Nova Biomedical
200 Prospect St.,
Waltham, Mass. 02254-9141
(617)894-0800

Organon Teknika
PO Box 99,
Jessup, Md. 20794
(800)638-7010

Orion Research
840 Memorial Dr.,
Cambridge, Mass. 02139
(800)225-1480

Ortho Diagnostic Systems
Route 202,
Raritan, N.J. 08869
(800)631-5807

Phytec
PO Box 724,
Huntingdon Valley, Pa. 19006
(800)742-8880
In Pennsylvania (215)938-0450

Quidel
11077 N. Torrey Pines Rd.,
La Jolla, Calif. 92037
(800)874-1517
In California (800)228-7704
(619)450-1533

Roche Diagnostic Systems
340 Kingsland St.,
Nutley, N.J. 07110
(800)631-0160

Sclavo Inc.
5 Mansard Ct.,
Wayne, N.J. 07470
(800)526-5260

SenTech Medical Corp.
3771 Lexington Ave. No.,
Arden Hills, Minn. 55112
(800)527-5577
In Minnesota (612)481-1000

Sequoia-Turner Corp.
755 Ravendale Dr.,
Mountain View, Calif. 94043
(800)227-8853
In California (800)982-6117
(415)969-5533

Seragen Diagnostics, Inc.
PO Box 1210,
Indianapolis, Ind. 46206
(800)428-4072
In Indiana (317)266-2924

SmithKline Diagnostics
PO Box 61947,
Sunnyvale, Calif. 94086
(800)538-1581
In California (408)732-6000

Streck Laboratories
14306 Industrial Rd.,
Omaha, Nebr. 68137
(800)228-6090
In Nebraska (402)333-1982

Syntex Medical Diagnostics
3300 Hillview Ave.,
Palo Alto, Calif. 94304
(415)494-1086

Technicon Instruments
511 Benedict Ave.,
Tarrytown, N.Y. 10591
(800)431-1970

Turpen Laboratory Systems
1650 Oak St.,
Lakewood, N.J.
(201)364-7600

Ulster Scientific, Inc.
PO Box 902,
Highland, N.Y. 12528
(800)431-8233
In New York (800)522-2257

Ventrex Laboratories
217 Read St.,
Portland, Me. 04103
(800)341-0463
In Maine (207)773-7231

V-Tech, Inc.
711 Forbes Ave.,
Pittsburgh, Pa. 15219
(412)562-8300

Wampole Laboratories
Half Acre Road,
Cranbury, N.J. 08512
(800)257-9525
In New Jersey (609)655-1100

Wellcome Diagnostics
3030 Cornwallis Rd.,
Research Park, N.C. 27709
(800)334-8570
In North Carolina (919)248-4617

Index

*Italic page numbers denote tabular material.

serum immunoassay for, 227-228

slide tests for urinary, 226, 230

specificity of tests for, 225

standardization of assays, 225

tube test for urinary, 226-227

Hyperaldosteronism, 66

Hyperglycemia, 59

Hypertension, 65-69

Hyperthyroidism, 66

Hyperventilation, 36

Hypoalbuminemia, 90

Hypoglycemia, 29

I

Idaho regulation, 113, 116

Identification of specimens, 130

IgA, *34*, 41, 42

IgG, *34*, 42

IgM, *34*, 41, 42

Immunization of staff, 158

Immunoassay, 22
for hCG, 227-228, 229-230

Immunofluorescence, 62

Immunoglobulins, 42

Immunohematology, 273

Incinerator, electric, 199, 207, 210

Incubator, 199, 207, 210
maintenance of, 264

Independent laboratories, 120, 122, 173 (*see also* Reference laboratories)

Indole, 205

Infection prevention, 158-159

Infectious mononucleosis (IM) tests, 230-233

In-service education, 133-134

Interest, 138

Interpretation of results, 39-47, 130-131

Iron, *34*, 35, 102

K

Ketone bodies, 55

Kodak chemistry system, 187

L

Laboratory (*see also* Independent laboratories; Reference laboratories)
amenities of, 148-149, 154
cabinets in, 147
expenses of, 137-141
location of, 145
safety of, 149-150, 155-160, 286
setting up of, 145-150
size of, 145-146
toilets in, 146
utilities in, 147-148

Laboratory testing loop, 5-7

Labor costs, 138

Lactate dehydrogenase (LD, LDH), 33, *34*, 42, 99-100, 187

Laparoscopy, 76

Laparotomy, 76

Legal considerations, of office laboratory, 287

Leucocyte esterase, 73, 105, 217

Leucocytes, 30

Liability risk, 125-135
don'ts, 134-135
in-service education, 133-134
interpretation of results, 130-131
process control, 129
records, 131-133
test reporting, 130

Licensing, of reference laboratory, 293, 297

Licensing laws, 111, 113, *114-115*, 116, 153, 283

Lipids, 42, 44

Lymphocytes, 70, 71

M

MacConkey agar, 205

Magnesium, *34*